Deep Learning for ECG Synthesis

Brian M. Hartz

One of the major causes of death is cardiovascular diseases. In 2019, it reached 32% of all deaths worldwide. ECG is widely used in the diagnosis of cardiovascular diseases mostly since it is non-invasive and painless. Diagnosis is usually performed by human specialists which is time-consuming and prone to human error, in case of availability. However, automatic ECG diagnosis is becoming increasingly more acceptable since not only it eliminates randomized human errors, but also it can be available as a bedside testing any time and anywhere using common and affordable wearable heart monitoring devices. Automatic ECG diagnosis algorithms are usually deep neural network classifier models which classify the ECG beats depending on the general pattern of the ECG heartbeat.

Electrocardiogram (ECG) datasets used for training the diagnosis classifiers, tend to be highly class-imbalanced due to the scarcity of abnormal cases and the abundance of normal cases. As such, the classifiers trained on class-imbalanced datasets usually perform poorly, especially on minor classes.

Additionally, the use of real patients' ECGs is highly regulated due to *privacy* issues. Therefore, there is always a need for more ECG data. One approach is to generate realistic synthetic ECG signals using Generative Adversarial Networks (GAN) to augment class-imbalanced datasets. The data generated by generative algorithms are not duplicates of the real training data and are unique for distinct latent variables, as generative algorithms map variables from latent space to the real space.

First Project: We studied the capability of generating synthetic ECG signals for 5 different models from the unconditional GAN family and compared their performances, focusing only on *Normal* cardiac cycles (monoclass). Dynamic Time Warping (DTW), Fréchet, and Euclidean distance functions were employed to quantitatively measure the *quality* of the generated beats. The *quality* of a beat signifies the existence of morphological patterns in a beat. We proposed and applied five different methods (metrics) for evaluating generated beats. The results show that all the tested models can, to some extent, successfully mass-generate acceptable heartbeats with high similarity in morphological features, and potentially all of them can be used to augment imbalanced datasets. However, visual inspections of generated beats favor BiLSTM-DC GAN and WGAN, as they produce statistically more acceptable beats. Also, with regards to the productivity rate metric, the Classic GAN is superior with a 72% productivity rate. We also designed a simple experiment with the state-of-the-art classifier (ECGResNet34) to show empirically that the augmentation of the imbalanced dataset by synthetic ECG signals could significantly improve the classification performance. This study is different from its predecessors as it includes WGAN and uses the *MLII* lead, which had not been done before. This paper has been published in *PLOS ONE* journal.

Second Project: We combined conditional GAN with WGAN-GP and developed AC-WGAN-GP in *1D form* for the first time to be applied to the MIT-BIH Arrhythmia dataset. We investigated the impact of data augmentation on arrhythmia classification. Two models were employed for ECG generation: *(i)* unconditional GAN; Wasserstein GAN with gradient penalty (WGAN-GP) trained on each class individually, and *(ii)* conditional GAN; one single Auxiliary Classifier WGAN-GP (AC-WGAN-GP) model trained on all classes and then used to generate synthetic beats in all classes. Two scenarios were defined for each case: *(a)* unscreened; i.e., all the generated synthetic beats were used, and *(b)* screened; i.e., only high-quality beats are selected and used, based on their Dynamic Time Warping (DTW) distance to a designated approved template. The state-of-the-art ResNet classifier (EcgResNet34) was trained on each of the four aforementioned study cases (augmented datasets), and the standard classification performance metrics (precision/recall/F1-Score micro- and macro-averaged, confusion matrices, multiclass precision-recall curves) were compared with those of the original imbalanced case. We also used a simple metric called *Net*

Improvement. All three metrics consistently show that unconditional GAN with raw generated data creates the best improvements. This paper has been presented and published in *IEEE BIBM Conference*, Las Vegas, 2022.

Third Project: We employed Diffusion models to generate synthetic ECG signals. Deep learning image processing models have had remarkable success in recent years in generating high-quality images. Particularly, the Improved Denoising Diffusion Probabilistic Models (DDPM) have shown superiority in image quality compared to state-of-the-art generative models, which motivated us to investigate its capability in generating synthetic electrocardiogram (ECG) signals. In this work, synthetic ECG signals are generated by the Improved DDPM and by the Wasserstein GAN with Gradient Penalty (WGANGP) models and then compared. To this end, we devised a pipeline to utilize DDPM in its original 2D form. First, the 1D ECG time series data is embedded into the 2D space, for which we employed the *Gramian Angular Summation/Difference Fields* (GASF/GADF) as well as *Markov Transition Fields* (MTF) to generate three 2D matrices from each ECG time series that, when put together, form a 3-channel 2D datum. Then, 2D DDPM is used to generate 2D 3-channel synthetic ECG images. The 1D ECG signals are reconstructed by de-embedding the 2D generated image files back into the 1D space. This work focuses on *unconditional* models and the generation of only *Normal sinus* ECG signals, where the Normal class from the MIT-BIH Arrhythmia dataset is used as the training phase. The quality, distribution, and the authenticity (equivalency) of the generated ECG signals by each model are compared. Our results show that, in the proposed pipeline, the WGAN-GP model is superior to DDPM by far in all the considered metrics consistently. This paper has been published in *IEEE Access* journal.

TABLE OF CONTENTS

Abstract v

List of Tables xv

List of Figures xvii

Chapter 1: Introduction 1

    1.1   Heart Disease Facts 1

    1.2   Cardiovascular System 1

        1.2.1   Blood Vessels 1

        1.2.2   Circulatory Systems 2

        1.2.3   Heart 3

        1.2.4   Heart's Conduction System 4

Chapter 2: Electrocardiogram (ECG) 8

    2.1   Introduction 8

    2.2   Cardiac Cycle 9

    2.3   Measuring ECG 10

        2.3.1   Bipolar Limb Leads 10

        2.3.2   Anatomical Planes and ECG Leads 10

Chapter 3: MIT-BIH Arrhythmia Dataset and Segmentation 12

    3.1   MIT-BIH Arrhythmia Dataset 12

    3.2   Data Description 12

    3.3   ECG Lead Configuration 13

    3.4   Digitization 13

3.5	Annotations	14
3.6	Patterns in Classes	17
3.7	class-imbalance in Dataset	18
3.8	Individual Beats as Time Series	18
3.9	Segmentation	18
	3.9.1 Pan-Tompkins Segmentation	18
	3.9.2 Window Segmentation	21
3.10	Resampling	22
3.11	Normalization	22
3.12	SMOTE Technique for class-imbalance	22

Chapter 4: Deep Generative Algorithms **24**

4.1	Introduction	24
4.2	Bayes Theorem	24
4.3	Variational Autoencoder	26
4.4	GAN	27
4.5	WGAN	28
4.6	WGAN-GP	30
4.7	Advantages and Issues of GAN Models	30
4.8	Conditional GAN	31
4.9	Denoising Diffusion Probabilistic Models	32
4.10	Improved DDPM	34
	4.10.1 Learned Sigma	34
	4.10.2 Noise Schedule	35
	4.10.3 Importance-sampled L_{vlb}	36

Chapter 5: Evaluation Metrics **38**

5.1	Introduction	38

5.2	Discriminative Models	38
5.3	Generative Models	39
5.4	Some Basic Concepts Used in Evaluation Metrics	40
5.5	Evaluation Metrics for Discriminative Models	40
	5.5.1 Confusion Matrix	40
	5.5.2 Overall Accuracy	41
	5.5.3 Precision	41
	5.5.4 Recall or Sensitivity	42
	5.5.5 F1-Score	42
	5.5.6 AUC-ROC	43
	5.5.7 AUC-PR	46
5.6	Evaluation Metrics for Generative Models	47
	5.6.1 Background	47
	5.6.2 Evaluation Pipeline	47
	5.6.3 Fidelity and Diversity	49
	5.6.4 Precision and Recall in Generative Models	50
5.7	Distance Functions or Similarity Measures	51
	5.7.1 Euclidean Distance	51
	5.7.2 Dynamic Time Warping (DTW)	52
	5.7.3 Fréchet Distance Measure	54
	5.7.4 Maximum Mean Discrepancy (MMD)	55
5.8	Metrics Used in This Study	57
	5.8.1 Quality: Average distance from an Approved Template	58
	5.8.2 Distributions	59
	5.8.3 Authenticity or Equivalency	59

Chapter 6: *(Paper 1)*

Synthetic ECG Signal Generation using Generative Neural Networks **63**

6.1	Motivation	63
6.2	Overview	64
6.3	Comparative Analysis to Previous Studies	64
6.4	Dataset and Segmentation	66
6.5	GAN Models	67
	6.5.1 Classic GAN (01)	67
	6.5.2 DC-DC GAN (02)	68
	6.5.3 BiLSTM-DC GAN (03)	69
	6.5.4 AE/VAE-DC GAN (04)	70
	6.5.5 WGAN (05)	73
	6.5.6 Hyperparameter Settings	74
6.6	Similarity Measures (Distance Functions)	75
	6.6.1 Dynamic Time Warping (DTW)	75
	6.6.2 Fréchet Distance Function	76
	6.6.3 Euclidean Distance Function	76
6.7	Templates	77
	6.7.1 Statistically Averaged Beat Template	77
	6.7.2 Expert-Eye Selected Template	78
6.8	and Evaluating the Generated Beats	78
	6.8.1 Method 1	78
	6.8.2 Method 2	79
	6.8.3 Method 3	80
	6.8.4 Method 4	81
	6.8.5 Method 5	82
	6.8.6 Authenticity or Equivalency Test	83
6.9	Platform and Code	84
6.10	Results and Discussion	84

6.10.1 Templates and Typical Normal Beat	84
6.10.2 Generated Beats by Different Models	85
6.10.3 Distance and Loss Functions	88
6.10.4 Performance Metrics	88
6.10.5 Authenticity Test and Efficacy of Augmentation	89
6.11 Conclusion	90
6.12 Future Works	92

Chapter 7: *(Paper 2)*
Arrhythmia Classification Using CGAN-Augmented ECG Signals — 93

7.1 Overview and Contribution	93
7.2 GAN Models	94
7.2.1 WGAN-GP (Unconditional)	94
7.2.2 AC-WGAN-GP (Conditional)	95
7.3 Dataset and Segmentation	95
7.4 Designs of Models	95
7.5 Experimental Description	99
7.5.1 Templates	100
7.5.2 Platform and Codes	100
7.6 Results and Discussion	101
7.6.1 Samples of Generated Beats	101
7.6.2 Precision or Recall	101
7.6.3 Quality of Generated Beats	102
7.6.4 Classification Results and Confusion Matrices	103
7.6.5 Net Improvements in True Positives	110
7.7 Conclusion	110

Chapter 8: *(Paper 3)*

Generation of Synthetic ECG Signals using Probabilistic Diffusion Models 112

8.1 Overview and Contribution 112

8.2 Proposed Pipeline 113

8.3 1D →2D Embedding 113

8.4 Polar Coordinate Representation of ECG 114

8.5 Gramian Angular Fields (GASF/GADF) 115

8.6 Markov Transition Fields (MTF) 116

8.7 2D →1D De-embedding 116

8.8 Precision or Recall 117

8.9 Area Under Precision-Recall Curve (AUC Pr-Re) 117

8.10 Area Under Receiver Operator Curve (AUC ROC) 117

8.11 Authenticity or Equivalency of Generated Beats 117

    8.11.1 Classifier: ECGResNet34 119

8.12 Experimental Setup 119

    8.12.1 WGAN-GP Model Design 119

    8.12.2 Improved DDPM Model Design 120

    8.12.3 Platform and GitHub Code 120

    8.12.4 DM, GAN and Real Study Cases 121

8.13 Results 121

    8.13.1 Quality 121

    8.13.2 Distribution 123

    8.13.3 Authenticity or Equivalency 124

8.14 Discussion 125

8.15 Conclusion 127

    8.15.1 what we did 127

    8.15.2 Why we did it 127

    8.15.3 How we did it 128

    8.15.4 results summary 128

  8.16 Limitations and Future Works 129

Chapter 9: Future Directions 130

  9.1 Diffusion-GAN Hybrid Model 130

  9.2 Cryo-ET/EM 131

LIST OF TABLES

3.1	Beat Annotations	15
3.2	Rhythm Annotations	16
3.3	Signal Quality and Comment Annotations	16
4.1	Bayesian Statistics Glossary	25
6.1	Comparison with Major Related Works - I	65
6.2	Comparison with Major Related Works - II	65
6.3	Comparison with Major Related Works - III	66
6.4	Classic GAN (01)	68
6.5	DC-DC GAN (02)	68
6.6	BiLSTM-DC GAN (03)	70
6.7	AE/VAE-DC GAN (04)	72
6.8	WGAN (05)	73
6.9	Method 1 (Portions of the Two Sets Compared with each other)	79
6.10	Method 2 (All Beats Compared with One Template, Averages)	80
6.11	Method 3 (Best Generated beat - Minimum Distance Functions)	81
6.12	Method 4 (Productivity - Percent of Acceptable Beats, above threshold)	82
6.13	Classification Report, Real Data, Balanced	90
6.14	Classification Report, Real Data, Imbalanced	90
6.16	Confusion Matrices (all values are in %)	90
6.15	Classification Report, Augmented Data, Balanced	91
7.1	Unconditional GAN Architecture	96
7.2	Conditional GAN Architecture - Generator	97
7.3	Conditional GAN Architecture - Critic	98
7.4	Selected Classes From MIT-BIH Arrhythmia Dataset Number of Samples	99

7.5	Quality of Generated Beats & Real Data Average DTW Distance from Template	102
7.6	Classification Report Reference Case (Imbalanced Dataset)	104
7.7	Confusion Matrix (%) Reference Case (Imbalanced Dataset)	104
7.8	Classification Report *Case I*: Conditional GAN, Raw Gen. Beats	105
7.9	Confusion Matrix (%) *Case I*: Conditional GAN, Raw Gen. Beats	105
7.10	Classification Report *Case II*: Conditional GAN, Screened Gen. Beats	106
7.11	Confusion Matrix (%) *Case II*: Conditional GAN, Screened Gen. Beats	106
7.12	Classification Report *Case III*: Unconditional GAN, Raw Gen. Beats	107
7.13	Confusion Matrix (%) *Case III*: Unconditional GAN, Raw Gen. Beats	107
7.14	Classification Report *Case IV*: Unconditional GAN, Screened	108
7.15	Confusion Matrix (%) *Case IV*: Unconditional GAN, Screened	108
7.16	Net Improvement in True Positives (%)	110
8.1	Authenticity or Equivalency Test — Training Set Supports	118
8.2	WGAN-GP Building Blocks	119
8.3	WGAN-GP Architecture	120
8.4	DM Case Studies	121
8.5	Quality of Generated Beats	123
8.6	MMD Value of Synthetic and Real Beats	123
8.7	Authenticity of Generated Beats	124
8.8	Confusion Matrices (all values are in %)	125

LIST OF FIGURES

1.1	Pulmonary and Systemic Circulation	2
1.2	Microcirculation Systems	3
1.3	Pericardium	4
1.4	Blood Flow Pathways	4
1.5	Electrical System of Heat	5
2.1	Moving Dipole	8
2.2	Chest Leads	11
2.3	Limb Leads	11
3.1	Morphological Patterns in Different Classes	17
3.2	MIT-BIH Arrhythmia Dataset Class Statistics	18
3.3	Pan-Tompkins Block Diagram [23]	19
3.4	Pan-Tompkins Flow Diagram [23]	20
3.5	Segmentation	21
4.1	Adversarial Training	28
4.2	DDPM with *Linear* (top) and *Cosine* (bottom) Noise Schedules	35
4.3	Variation of $\bar{\alpha}_t$ with time steps in *linear* and *cosine* schedules	35
5.1	Confuision Matrix- Monoclass	41
5.2	Confusion Matrix - Multiclass	41
5.3	AUC ROC	44
5.4	AUC PR - Monoclass	47
5.5	AUC PR - Multiclass	47
5.6	Dynamic Time Warping [87]	53
5.7	ResNet Building Block [35]	60

5.8	Example network architectures for ImageNet.	62
6.1	GAN Models Used	67
6.2	Model 01	67
6.3	Model 02 (Generator)	69
6.4	Model 02 (Discriminator)	69
6.5	Model 03	70
6.6	Model 04 (Generator)	72
6.7	Model 04 (Discriminator)	73
6.8	Model 05 (Generator)	74
6.9	Model 05 (Discriminator)	74
6.10	Statistically Averaged Template	77
6.11	Selected Template	78
6.12	Generated Beats, Classic GAN (01)	85
6.13	Generated Beats, DC-DC GAN (02)	86
6.14	Generated Beats, BiLSTM-DC GAN (03)	86
6.15	Generated Beats, AE/VAE-DC-DC GAN (04)	87
6.16	Generated Beats, WGAN (05)	87
6.17	DTW Similarity Measure and Loss Functions vs Epoch Numbers	88
7.1	Architecture of Developed $1D$ Conditional WGAN-GP	98
7.2	Samples of Generated Beats	101
7.3	Precision-Recall Curves	109
8.1	Proposed Pipeline	113
8.2	*Normal Sinus* ECG Beat in Cartesian and Polar Coordinates	115
8.3	Samples of Synthetically Generated ECG Signals	122
8.4	Precision-Recall Curves	126
9.1	Generative learning trilemma	130

9.2	Diffusion-GAN Hybrid Architecture	131
9.3	Cryo ET/EM Technology	132
9.4	Cryo ET/EM 3D Image Reconstruction	132

CHAPTER 1: INTRODUCTION

1.1 Heart Disease Facts

Heart disease is the leading cause of death and one person dies every 33 seconds from cardiovascular disease in the United States. Heart diseases cost the United States about $239.9 billion each year. Angioplasty, coronary bypass surgery, valve replacement, stenting, the implantation of pacemakers/defibrillators are currently routine treatment procedures [24, 41], [77].

1.2 Cardiovascular System

The principal components of the cardiovascular system are: *(1)* blood, *(2)* blood vessels, *(3)* heart and *(4)* lymphatic system (the tissues and organs that produce, store, and carry white blood cells that fight infections and other diseases).

1.2.1 Blood Vessels

Th human body exhibits an exceptional level of blood vessel branching, which assures nearly every cell in the body is within a short distance from at least one of the capillaries. Nutrients and metabolic products move between cells and capillary vessels by tissue fluid and diffusion. Further movement into the cells happen through diffusion and mediated transport by the specialized proteins across the cell membrane [41].

There are two closed-loop pathways in our blood vessels, both of which originate and return to the heart: *(1)* pulmonary circulation and *(2)* systemic circulation. The pulmonary circulation system is composed of right heart pump and the lungs. The Circulatory circulation system, on the other hand, consists of the left heart pump and supplies blood to the systemic organs (i.e., all the tissues and organs other than the gas exchange portion of the lungs).

The left and the right heart pumps function as two in-series pumps, therefore both circulate exactly the same flow rate and amount of blood throw the pulmonary and systemic systems.

1.2.2 Circulatory Systems

Systemic Circuit

Blood is discharged from the left ventricle through one single large artery: the *aorta*. Aorta is the largest artery in the body with a diameter of 20-30 mm from which all the other arteries of the systemic circulation branch. It progressively divide into smaller vessels. Blood moves from *arterioles* (small blood vessel branching from the arteries which are located between arteries and the capillaries) to the capillaries.

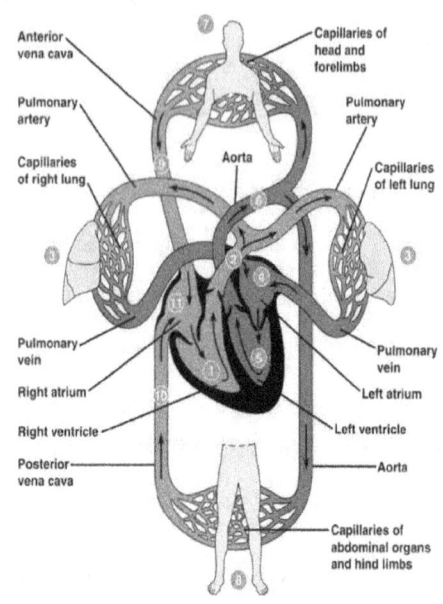

Figure 1.1: Pulmonary and Systemic Circulation

Capillaries are the smallest vessels in the human body (5-10 μm) with an estimated number of 10 billion in an average human body. The individual length of a capillary is around 1 mm and the total length of capillaries in an average adult human body is estimated as 25,000 miles. The thickness of most capillaries is just a little bit more than the thickness of single cell, which facilitates the capillaries main function: the exchange of materials (small molecules such as O2, CO2, sugar, amino acids and water) between cells and in the tissue and the blood.

Then, blood exits the capillaries and enters the venules. Venules are small blood vessels that collect deoxygenated blood from the capillaries and gradually merge into larger veins. Venules are located at the downstream end of the capillary network and serve as the bridge between capillaries and veins within the circulatory system. The flow of blood through arterioles, capillaries and venules, is called *Microcirculation* collectively. Blood starts its jouney back to the heart from venules which is the endpoint of the pulmonary circuit.

Smooth muscle fibers stimulate contractions and relaxations so as to regulate blood flow through the capillaries. Blood flows through capillaries intermittently (*vasomotion* as a result of periodic contraction of smooth muscles (5-10 times per minute). The periodic contraction of smooth muscles are regulated both by local chemical conditions (metabolically) and by sympathetic control.

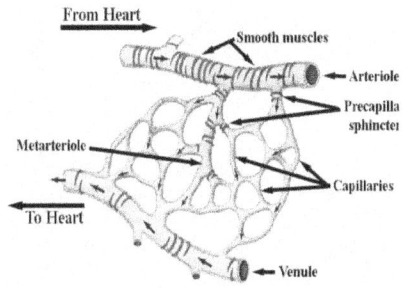

Figure 1.2: Microcirculation Systems

Pulmonary Circuit

Blood discharges from the right ventricle in a single large vessel, the pulmonary artery (trunk), which shortly (after a few centimeters) divides into two arteries, each supplying one lung. Arteries in the lungs divide into smaller arterioles and ultimately into capillaries which connects the two circulation circuits. As blood flows through the lung capillaries, it picks up oxygen which causes the hemoglobin in the red blood cells become loaded with oxygen. The oxygenated blood eventually enters the left atrium [41].

1.2.3 Heart

Human heart is a muscular pump which performs two main functions: *(1)* to collect blood from tissues of the body (systemic organs) and pump it to the lungs (pulmonary system) and *(2)* to collect blood from the lungs and pump it to all tissues of the body. The contraction of the cardiac muscle cells is trigered by the flow of Ca^{2+} into the cell. The free movement of ions between cells allows for the direct transmission of an electrical impulse through an entire network of cardiac muscle cells. This impulse creates a signal to all cells in the network to contract at the same time.

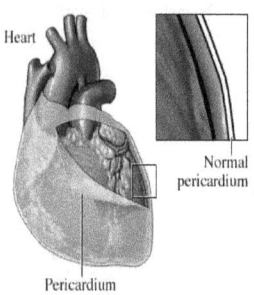

Figure 1.3: Pericardium

Figure 1.4: Blood Flow Pathways

Human heart is suspended in the thoracic cavity and lies in a fibrous sac known as *pericardium* (Fig. 1.3). The *pericardial fluid* inside the sac lubricates the surface of the heart and allows it to move freely during the contraction and relaxation.

There are 4 valves in the heart: the tricuspid valve, mitral valve, pulmonic valve, and aortic valve. The tricuspid and mitral valves are positioned between the atria and ventricles. The pulmonic and aortic valves are located between the ventricles and great vessels. The pathway of blood flow through the chambers of the heart is shown in Fig. 1.4. Venous deoxygenated blood, returning from the systemic organs, enters the right atrium through Superior Vena Cava (SVC) and Inferior Vena Cava (IVC). Then it passes through the *tricuspid valve* and enters the right ventricle, where it is pumped into the pulmonary artery through the pulmonary valve during the contraction. The oxygenated blood returns from the pulmonary capillary beds to the left atrium. Then, it passes through the mitral valve and enters the left ventricle from where it is pumped into the aorta and the systemic organs through the aortic valve [41].

Ventricles, which do the main pumping action, are closed chambers surrounded by muscular walls. Valves passively allow flow only in certain directions in reaction to the change of pressure change across them caused by contraction and relaxations in the heart muscles.

1.2.4 Heart's Conduction System

The main components of the conduction system are: *(1)* sinoatrial (SA) node, *(2)* atrioventricular (AV) node, *(3)* bundle of His, *(4)* right and left main bundle branches, *(5)* Purkinje fibers.

There are 2 main types of cardiac myocytes (muscle cells) in the myocardium: *(1)* Conducting Cells (Pacemaker Cells), *(2)* Contractile Cells (Non-Pacemaker Cells).

Pacemaker Cells

The heart has the ability to generate its own spontaneous electrical impulse without any external stimuli. This happens in the specialized myocytes in the myocardium that have the ability to generate spontaneous action potentials. These cells are located in the electrical pathways (the entire conduction system) of the heart. They generate and transmit electrical impulses throughout the myocardium. As the electrical impulse passes through the conduction system and the myocardium, it causes contraction in the muscles. The rate at which the pacemaker sends electrical signals is called the *Heart Rate*.

Contractile Cells

More than %99 of the myocytes are of contractile cells. The action potential which passes through the conduction system causes depolarization (contraction) in the contractile cells.

SA Node

In a normal functioning heart, the SA node is the starting point of the conducting system and is located in the right atrium near the superior vena cava entry and is comprised of many pacemaker cells. Unlike regular cardiac muscle cells, pacemaker cells have the ability to generate electrical impulses spontaneously without external stimulation at a rate of 60-100 beats per minute (sinus rhythm).

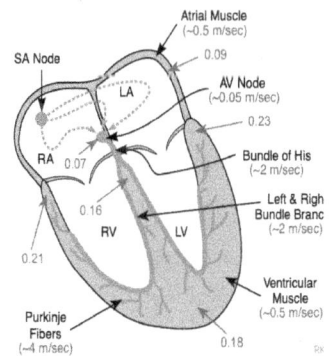

Figure 1.5: Electrical System of Heat

Depolarization in SA Node

- **Resting State:** The SA node starts in a state of electrical rest, known as the resting membrane potential. At this stage, the inside of the cells has a negative charge compared to the outside (polarized). This resting membrane potential is maintained by the movement of ions across the cell membrane, mainly through ion channels.

- **Spontaneous Depolarization:** During the spontaneous depolarization phase, a slow influx of sodium ions (Na^+) occurs, which gradually reduces the negative charge inside the cells and brings them closer to the threshold for firing an action potential.

- **Threshold Potential:** As the membrane potential of the SA node cells reaches a certain threshold level, it triggers the opening of voltage-gated calcium channels (Ca^{2+}). These channels allow an influx of calcium ions into the cells, initiating a rapid depolarization phase.

- **Rapid Depolarization:** The influx of calcium ions causes a rapid and significant change in the membrane potential, shifting it from negative to positive. This electrical depolarization spreads across the SA node cells, generating an action potential.

Repolarization in SA Node

- **Inactivation of Calcium Channels:** Once the membrane potential reaches its peak positive value during depolarization, the voltage-gated calcium channels responsible for the influx of calcium ions begin to close, reducing the flow of calcium ions into the cells.

- **Potassium Ion Efflux:** As the calcium channels close, voltage-gated potassium channels open, allowing potassium ions (K^+) to flow out of the cells. This potassium efflux helps restore the negative charge inside the cells, leading to repolarization.

- **Resting State Restoration:** The movement of potassium ions out of the cells brings the membrane potential back to its negative resting state. The sodium-potassium pump, an enzyme present in the cell membrane, actively transports sodium ions (Na^+) out of the cell and potassium ions (K^+) back in, further contributing to the restoration of the resting state.

The generated plus in the SA node travels towards the AV node through the 3 intra-atrial pathways conduction tracts which are bands of specialised myocytes. The action potential depolarize and contracts the atria as it travels through the atria, which pushes the blood into the ventricles during the *diastole*. Atrial depolarization (contraction) is represented on ECG by the P-wave. The action potential travels to the left atrium via *Bachmann's bundle*.

AV Node

The action potential converges into another node, called atrioventricular (AV) node node, after passing through the 3 pathways. The AV node is located at the base of the right atrium, near the atrioventricular septum (Fig. 1.5). Some of the functions of the AV node consist of:

- The AV node is responsible for delaying the electrical signal that travels from the atria to the ventricles. Since the electrical impulse travels faster than the blood flow, this delay allows the atria to contract and complete their pumping action before the ventricles receive the electrical signal, ensuring efficient blood flow.

- Transmission of the electrical impulses from atria to the ventricles.

- The AV node helps regulate the heart rate by controlling the number of electrical impulses that reach the ventricles. It acts as a gatekeeper, allowing only a certain number of impulses to pass through to maintain an appropriate heart rate and prevent excessive or irregular heartbeats.

The depolarization proceeds through the bundle of His, which is located in the *triangle of Koch*, along with the AV node. The depolarization spreads to both the left and the right bundle branches, after leaving the bundle of His. The bundles carry the depolarization to the left and right ventricles, respectively. the impulse travels through the remainder of the Purkinje fibers through which the ventricular myocardial depolarization spreads.

CHAPTER 2: ELECTROCARDIOGRAM (ECG)

2.1 Introduction

Electrocardiogram (ECG) or EKG (in German: Electrokardiogram), reportedly first recorded in 1903 by Willem Einthoven, is a cumulative measure of electrical activity of the heart changes versus time as the action potentials propagate through the heart during each cardiac cycle. It shows the *overall* electrical differences across the heart when individual atrial and ventricular cells go through depolarization/repolarization process.

For the purpose of ECG the human body can be considered as a very large conductor filled tissues (such as the heart) surrounded by conductive ionic fluid. As the action potentials pass through the heart muscles and creates contractions (depolarized), the rest of the myocardia are at rest (polarized), therefore, a moving charge separation or dipole wavefront is formed in the heart (Fig. 2.1), which creates a fluctuating current flow across the heart and the body which can be detected and picked up by the electrodes attached to the surface of the body. The intensity of the induced voltage in the electrode depends on the orientation of the electrodes with respect to the net moving dipole. obviously, any movement in the body of the subject, would be accompanied by some electrical activity in the skeletal muscles, which would contribute to the voltages detected by the electrode on the surface of the patient. So it's of crucial importance that the patient is essentially motionless during the ECG recording.

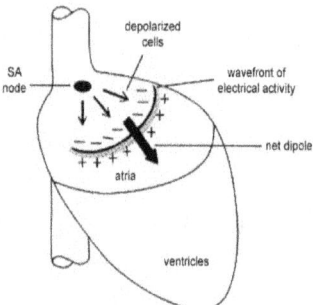

Figure 2.1: Moving Dipole

2.2 Cardiac Cycle

Cardiac Cycle has two phases: *(1)* Diastole and *(2)* Systole.

Diastole (from Greek *diastolē*: dilation) refers to the phase of the cardiac cycle when the heart muscles (particularly ventricles) is relax and expand, allowing the chambers of the heart to fill with blood. In diastole, the ventricles are relaxed and at low pressure state. The atria begin to fill with blood and the pressure in atria begin to rise. Eventually, when it exceeds the pressure in ventricle, the valve will open and let the blood flow to the ventricles. Up to this point no contraction has been taken place and the blood flows passively.

When the ventricles are filled with blood, the pressure approaches the atrial pressure and the blood flow slows down. Now the contraction takes place in the atria so that the blood flow can continue.

The cardiac cycle begins with firing of SA node in the right atrium. This firing is not detected in ECG because its amplitude is too weak to be detected. However, the contraction (depolarization) of the atria, which is strong enough, is captured in ECG as the *P-wave*. The *P-wave* duration is around 80-100 ms. After the end of the *P-wave* and while the ECG signal returns to the baseline, the action potential spread into the AV node and the bundle of His, which is not detectable again because there are not too many cells to amplify the depolarization. Then the right and left ventricles begin to depolarize which lead to the recordable QRS complex. It lasts about 100 ms in duration. First there's a negative deflection, *Q-wave*, then the strong positive deflection, *R-wave*, which is followed by the second negative deflection, *S-wave*. At the end of QRS complex, the contraction of the ventricles are finished and the signal returns to the baseline. Simultaneous to the QRS complex, the atria repolarize (relax), however, it is sufficiently masked by the much stronger QRS complex (outnumbered by the large tissues in the ventricles). At the end of the QRS complex the signal returns to the baseline and the ventricles repolarize (relax) which is detected as the *T-wave*. *T-wave* is the last potential detected in a cardiac cycle.

It is obvious from the normal ECG signal that the QRS complex has a much stronger (higher) and shorter duration peak than the *P-* or *T-waves*. It is because much bigger cardiac tissue (larger number of myocytes) participate in the ventricular depolarization simultaneously, and also because of the heart physiology, the ventricular contraction is much more synchronized than either atrial depolarization or ventricular repolarization.

In some individuals, there is a *U-wave* also present in the ECG which is believed to be the effect of repolarization of the Purkinje system.

2.3 Measuring ECG

When two electrodes are placed on the surface of the human skin and the potential difference between them is monitored, the measured potential is affected by the net effect of the depolarization and repolarization of nearly 300 billion cardiomyocytes in the heart. The detected waveform features depend not only on the amount of the cardiac tissue involved, but also on the orientation of the electrodes with respect to the major dipoles in the heart.

2.3.1 Bipolar Limb Leads

Electrodes are the pads that are put on the patient's skin, however, an ECG *lead* is a graphical representation of the electrical activity of the heart. I fact leads are calculated using the information provided by the electrodes. The standard ECG has 12 leads which are collected using 10 electrodes. These 12 leads are divided into *limb leads* and *chest leads* or *pericordial leads*.

All the 12 leads in a standard ECG measure the same electrical activity, however, from different angle and projected to different planes.

2.3.2 Anatomical Planes and ECG Leads

ECG projects the net effect of the electrical activity of the heart onto various planes, namely, the horizontal and the vertical (frontal) planes. The placement of the electrodes (configuration) determines which plane is being projected to. The reference electrode is usually put on the right ankle. The potential difference between any electrode and the reference electrode is the projection on the frontal plane. On the other hand, the potential difference between the electrode on the

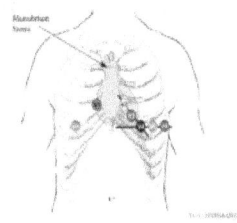
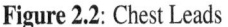
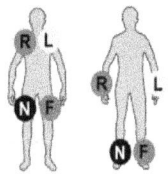

Figure 2.2: Chest Leads   **Figure 2.3**: Limb Leads

sternum and the electrode placed on the back at the level, produces the projection of the same electrical activity onto the horizontal plane.

There are 6 limb leads (Fig. 2.3): I, II, III, aVF, aVR and aVL (derived from only three electrodes placed on right arm, left arm and left leg) capture the projections of the electrical vectors on the frontal plane. The chest (pericordial) leads, i.e., $V1$, $V2$, $V3$, $V4$, $V5$, $V6$ are located anteriorly on the chest. The standard placement of the chest leads involves placing them on specific anatomical landmarks on the anterior chest wall. Their reference point is inside the chest, i.e., the Wilson's central terminal (WCT). The WCT is a virtual reference point that is calculated using the average of the voltages from the limb leads (I, II, and III, the original Einthoven leads) and is used as a reference for the chest leads. [20].

CHAPTER 3: MIT-BIH ARRHYTHMIA DATASET AND SEGMENTATION

3.1 MIT-BIH Arrhythmia Dataset

The dataset used in this study is the MIT-BIH Arrhythmia Database [27], [53]. It is well-known and widely used collection of data for studying arrhythmia. This dataset is a product of laboratories at *Boston's Beth Israel Hospital* (now the Beth Israel Deaconess Medical Center) and also at Massachusetts Institute of Technology (MIT). They started to collect data from patients in 1975 distributed their product in 1980. This database is historically the very first standard dataset for testing and evaluation of arrhythmia detectors which was made publicly available. It also has been widely used for basic cardiac analysis, with more than 3700 citations as of today. It was originally distributed on 9-track half-inch digital tape at 800 and 1600 bpi and also on quarter-inch IRIG-format FM analog tape [27]. The CD-ROM format of the database was published in 1989.

3.2 Data Description

There are 48 30-min selection of two-channel ambulatory recordings in the digitized MIT-BIH Arrhythmia Data base [27]. The data were collected between 1975 and 1979 from 47 subjects at the BIH Arrhythmia Laboratory. From the 48 recording in the dataset, 23 were chosen randomly (using a random number table) from a set of 4000 24-hour ambulatory ECG Holter recording (60% from inpatients and 40% from outpatients). This group is intended to serve as an unbiased representative sample from routine clinical use which contain various waveforms and artifacts that an arrhythmia detector can detect.

The remaining 25 recordings were selected from the same set, however, the selection was not random; only those recordings were targeted that included some sort of less common but clinically significant arrhythmias. Such anomalies are very hard to come by in a randomly selected recordings, e.g., complex ventricular, junctional and supra-ventricular arrhythmias and conduction anomalies.

The analog data were recorded using Del Mar Avionics model 445 two channel Holter recorders, whereas for digitization, a Del Mar Avionics model 660 unit is used to playback the recordings.

The digitization of the recordings were done for each channel at the frequency of 360 Hz with 11-bit resolution over a 10 mV range. Two cardiologists annotated the recordings and labeled each beat independently and any discrepancy was resolved by consensus, so that one reference set of annotations were provided and included with the dataset which can be read by computer easily.

3.3 ECG Lead Configuration

The upper signal in most records is a *modified limb lead II (MLII)*, the electrode of which is placed on the chest. The lower signal usually is a *modified lead V1 (sometimes V2 or V5 or V4)*. These electrodes also are placed on the chest. Normal QRS complex is more prominent usually in the upper signal. The lead axis for the lower signal may be nearly orthogonal to the mean cardiac electrical axis, however (i.e., normal beats are usually biphasic and may be nearly isoelectric) [52]. Therefore, *Normal Sinus Beats* are usually more difficult to recognize in the lower signal while ectopic beats will often more prominent in the lower signal. One notable point is that the signals in the record 114 are reversed.

3.4 Digitization

The analog signals in the recordings are filtered using a band-pass filter to limit analog-to-digital converter saturation and for-anti-aliasing. The pass-band was from 0.1 to 100 Hz, which was well beyond the limit frequencies recoverable from recordings. The filtered data were digitized at 360 Hz, which facilitates the implementation of *digital notch filter* in the detectors. Since the mains frequency was 60 Hz and the recorders were battery-powered, most of the 60 Hz noise presented in the recordings came from the playback.

3.5 Annotations

The annotation process started off with preparation of a preliminary set of labels produced by a simple slope-sensitive QRS detector, which allowed to identify Normal Sinus Beats easily. For each 30-minute record two 150-ft chart recordings were printed with the preliminary labels were printed on the margin. Two cardiologist worked on labeling and annotating the beats independently, who corrected errors and added any missed labels. The correction then were transcribed and analyzed by an auditing program. Any inconsistency between the two cardiologist's labels, were resolved by consensus between the two cardiologists.

The labels on manually labeled signals were not always located on the R-peak exactly, as opposed to the automatically labeled ones. This should be kept in mind and if it affects any research, the locations of the labels should be corrected manually, as we did in this research.

The database contains nearly 109,000 beats. In general there are three types of annotations in the database:

- Beat annotations:
    - where the type of the beat is determined and labeled
- Rhythm Annotations:
    - appear below the level used for beat annotations which explain about the rhythm rather than the pattern in each individual beat
- Signal quality
    - appear above the level used for beat annotations and explain about the signal quality

	Beat Annotations
. or N	Normal Beat
L	Left bundle branch block beat
R	Right bundle branch block beat
A	Atrial premature beat
a	Aberrated atrial premature beat
J	Nodal (junctional) premature beat
S	Supraventricular premature beat
V	Premature ventricular contraction
F	Fusion of ventricular and normal beat
[	Start of ventricular flutter/fibrillation
!	Ventricular flutter wave
]	End of ventricular flutter/fibrillation
e	Atrial escape beat
j	Nodal (junctional) escape beat
E	Ventricular escape beat
/	Paced beat
f	Fusion of paced and normal beat
x	Non-conducted P-wave (blocked APB)
Q	Unclassifiable beat
|	Isolated QRS-like artifact

Table 3.1: Beat Annotations

Rhythm Annotations (appear below beat annotation level)	
(AB	Atrial bigeminy
(AFIB	Atrial fibrillation
(AFL	Atrial flutter
(B	Ventricular bigeminy
(BII	2° heart block
(IVR	Idioventricular rhythm
(N	Normal sinus rhythm
(NOD	Nodal (A-V junctional) rhythm
(P	Paced rhythm
(PREX	Pre-excitation (WPW)
(SBR	Sinus bradycardia
(SVTA	Supraventricular tachyarrhythmia
(T	NVentricular trigeminy
(VFL	Ventricular flutter
(VT	Ventricular tachycardia

Table 3.2: Rhythm Annotations

Signal Quality and Comment Annotations (appear above beat annotation level)	
qq	Signal quality change: the first character ('c' or 'n') indicates the quality of the upper signal (clean or noisy), and the second character indicates the quality of the lower signal
U	Extreme noise or signal loss in both signals: ECG is unreadable
M (or MISSB)	Missed Beat
P (or PSE)	Pause
T (or TS)	Tape slippage

Table 3.3: Signal Quality and Comment Annotations

3.6 Patterns in Classes

The morphological patterns in MIT-BIH Arrhythmia Data set is shown in Figure 3.1. These are individual beat after segmenting the continuous 30-min ECG signals. They are also re-sampled to a fixed length of 256 samples per beat. The morphological patterns exhibit clear distinctions from one another, indicating that a classifier can easily differentiate them easily.

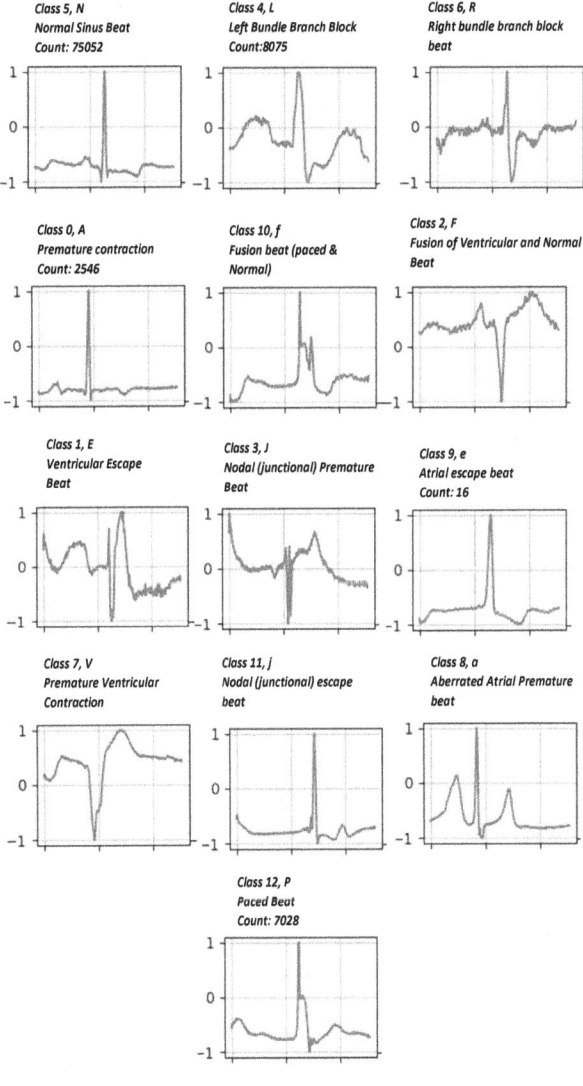

Figure 3.1: Morphological Patterns in Different Classes

3.7 class-imbalance in Dataset

Figure 3.2 shows the statistics in MIT-BIH Arrhythmia dataset. The dataset, similar to most ECG datasets, is heavily skewed towards class N, which constitutes 68.5% of the data. This is due to the abundance of normal patients and normal beats and the scarcity of the abnormal cases.

Class	Class	Count	%
5	N	75052	68.5
4	L	8075	7.3
6	R	7259	6.6
7	V	7130	6.5
12	/	7028	6.4
0	A	2546	2.3
10	f	982	0.9
2	F	803	0.7
11	j	229	0.2
8	a	150	0.1
1	E	106	0.1
3	J	83	0.1
15	Q	33	0.0
9	e	16	0.0
14	S	2	0.0
	Σ	109,494	

Figure 3.2: MIT-BIH Arrhythmia Dataset Class Statistics

3.8 Individual Beats as Time Series

Each individual beat is in fact a time series, i.e., a one-dimensional vector representing the progression of the voltage on a particular electrode over time. The actual dataset is saved as set of vectors, which, when plotted would look like patterns shown in Figure 3.1.

3.9 Segmentation

3.9.1 Pan-Tompkins Segmentation

Pan-Tompkins (PT) algorithm [23, 58] is an algorithm developed by Jiapu Pan (Shanghai Second Medical College) and Willis J. Tompkins (University of Wisconsin, Madison) in 1985 to detect the QRS complex in ECG. The algorithm consist of different steps:

- Pre-processing
    - Noise removal
    - signal smoothing
    - width and QRS slope increasing
- Decision
    - using thresholds to select only the signal peaks and discard *noise* peaks

Fig. 3.3 shows the block flow diagram of PT algorithm. It consists of a band-pass (a low pass plus a high pass) filter, derivative, squaring function, Moving Window Integration (WMI) and decision making based on thresholds. The sampling rate used in this method is 200 Hz. Thresholds are adjusted automatically and dynamically to adapt to the changes in heart rate and in morphology in QRS complex.

Band-Pass Filter

A low-pass filter (LPF) and a high-pass filter (HPF) are cascaded to achieve a passband of 5 – 15 Hz. The LPF eliminates high-frequency noises (e.g., EMG (electrical signals) generated by nearby muscle contractions), power-line interference, T-wave interference) whereas HPF removes low-frequency noise such as baseline wandering. These filters are both real-time recursive filters in which poles are located to cancel zeros on the unit circle of the z-plane which result in a filter design with with integer coefficients.

Table 1: A Comparison between the NST and MIT databases

Characteristics	Databases	
	NST	MIT
Device Type	Hospital Holter	Hospital Holter
Signal Type	Ambulatory ECG	Ambulatory ECG
Record	12	48
Duration	30 minutes	
Activity Type	N/A	N/A
Noise	Artefacts in ambulatory ECG and motion artefact (from the physically active subject)	Artefacts in ambulatory ECG

The MIT database [15] has reportedly been used in many publications. This database includes 48 heartbeat recordings at 360 Hz. Each record of 47 different patients is 30 minutes in duration and contains two leads: 1) Lead A, modification of Lead II and; 2) Lead B, regular lead V1, V2, V5 or V4. The database has been employed by researchers to test algorithms for QRS detection and arrhythmia detection and classification [1]. As per Mood and Mark [16], Lead A is commonly used to identify the characteristics of heartbeats while Lead B is normally used to identify arrhythmic types Supraventricular ectopic beats and Ventricular ectopic beat.

2.3 Pan-Tompkins Algorithm

The Pan-Tompkins algorithm utilises the amplitude, slope, and width of an integrated window to identify the R-peaks in QRS complexes [12]. The algorithm consists of two stages, which are pre-processing and decision. In pre-processing, the raw ECG signal is prepared as input to the detection process. Pre-processing includes noise removal, signal smoothing, and width and QRS slope increasing. Then, the decision stage.

The algorithm consists of a band-pass filter (Low Pass and High Pass Filters), derivatives, a squaring function, a moving window integration (WMI), threshold, and decision, as shown in the diagram in Figure 2. The sampling rate of this method is 200 Hz. In this algorithm, the false detection filter. To adapt to the changes in QRS morphology and heart rate, the thresholds were automatically adjusted with the parameter in the decision stages. The detailed algorithm process flow is presented in the flowchart of Figure 3.

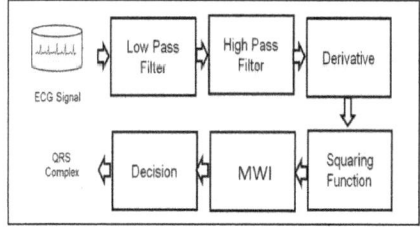

Figure 2: A block diagram of The Pan-Tompkins algorithm

Figure 3.3: Pan-Tompkins Block Diagram [23]

Derivative

At the derivative step, the ECG signal is differentiated, i.e., the slope information is determined. The low-frequency P and T waves are suppressed at this stage to get high-frequency signals existing in QRS complex [23].

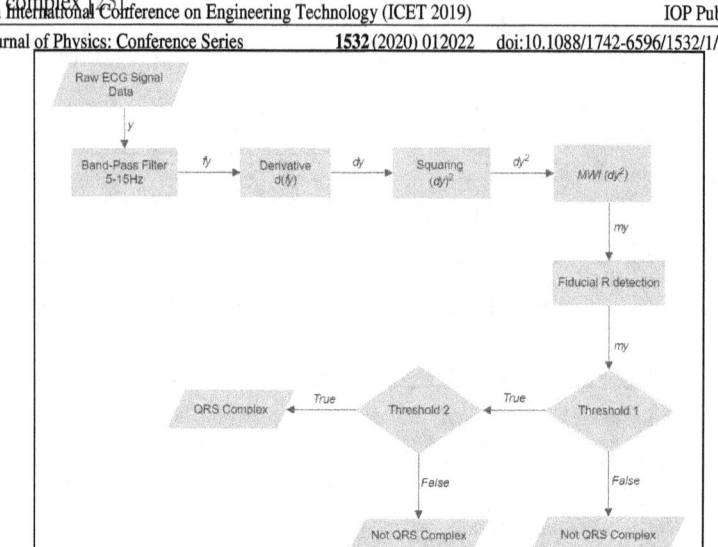

Figure 3. Pan-Tompkins Flow Diagram [23]

The explanations of each process are given with the output. These show the implementation of the algorithms using the NST database (Record 118e12) and the MIT database (Record 118). In Figure 2, the output of each process in the algorithm is presented. Since Record 118e12 (NST) with 12 dB SNR was produced from Record 118 (MIT), a comparison between both records of noisy and clean data can also be observed. A more detailed explanation of each process is given below [12].

Squaring Function

The squaring function assures all the values are positive. The higher amplitudes of QRS complex are enhanced even further compared to that of T-wave, which often cause false detection.

2.3.1 Band-Pass Filter

The band-pass filter reduces the influence of noise. The desirable passband maximises the QRS energy up to a suitable frequency. The Low Pass Filter (LPF) and High Pass Filter (HPF) were cascaded to achieve an approximately 5–15 Hz passband. LPF was used to remove the high-frequency noise such as EMG, Power Line Interference, and T-wave interference while allowing the low-frequency signals to be recorded. HPF was used to remove the low-frequency noise such as the Baseline Wander.

Moving Window Integration

The main purpose of Moving Window Integration (MWI) is to smooth the input signal and enhance the QRS complex. A window of 30 samples (150 ms) is used in PT algorithm as the sampling rate is 200 samples/sec.

Figures 4.1 and 4.2 show the raw ECG signal (a) and the output of the Band-Pass Filter process (b). Since NST data was added with the Motion Artefact noise, this data produced a lower quality ECG signal compared to the MIT data. The noise is illustrated in Figure 4.1(a) where the signal displays unstable amplitudes, which influenced the R-peak identification on the signal. However, the digital band-pass filter output shows that the Motion Artefact signal was improved and a better quality signal was produced after filtering, as shown in Figures 4.1(b) and 4.2 (b).

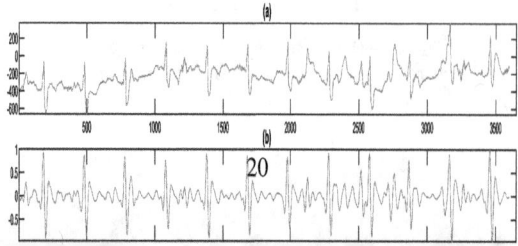

tion: breaking up the continuous multi-beat ECG signals
 ual single beats

ndow: R-peak, fixed number of timestep forward and backward
e window: RR distance, 75% forward - 75% backward

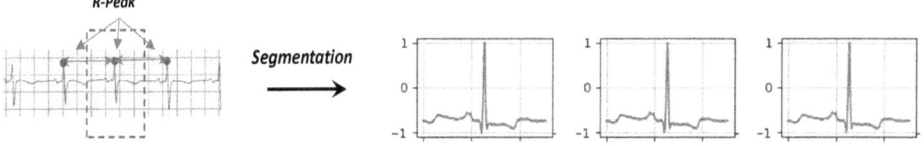

Figure 3.5: Segmentation

3.9.2 Window Segmentation

In this method, a cutoff window is defined and the beat is isolated from the continuous signal.

Fixed Window Segmentation

A *fixed number of timesteps* forward and backward of the R-peak is chosen as the cutoffs and the beat between them is saved as one single beat. In this method, if the hart rate changes, there would be a chance that the part of the beat is lost.

Adaptive Window Segmentation

The distance between the R-peak and the last and the next R-peaks are calculated, and 75% of each distance is taken as the cutoff limit, and the beat between them is saved as the beat. This method compensates for any change in the heart beat and no information would be lost because of that.

3.10 Resampling

After each beat of a record is saved, they are all resampled to 256 time step because the inputs should be of the same length in some deep learning models. This is done simply by the *scipy.signal.resample()* method.

3.11 Normalization

All the individual beats after segmentation and resampling, are normalized in the *amplitude* using the following formula [82]:

$$v_{normalized} = \frac{n-i}{n}\frac{v_i - v_{min}}{v_0 - v_{min}} + \frac{i}{n}\frac{v_i - v_{min}}{v_0 - vmin} \qquad (3.1)$$

Amplitude normalization, in fact, *unpersonalizes* the ECG beats, i.e., it enables the mixing of the beats from different patients, otherwise, the intensity of electrode voltages would make beats in the same class from different patient different.

3.12 SMOTE Technique for class-imbalance

A dataset is imbalanced if the classification categories are not approximately equally represented [14]. In fraud detection datasets, an imbalance of 100 to 1 is a norm, while some cases with a ration of 100, 000 to 1 have also reported [61].

Real-world datasets are usually and predominately composed of *normal* samples with only a small percentage of *abnormal* cases. Also, mostly, the cost of misclassifying an *abnormal* as a *normal* case is much higher than the reverse.

The machine learning community has addressed the class-imbalance isuue in two ways:

- Assigning distinct costs to training examples [60]

- Resampling the original dataset (oversampling the minority class and/or under-sampling the majority class)

SMOTE blends the under-sampling of the majority class with a special form of over-sampling the minority class [14]. In SMOTE technique, *synthetic* samples from the minority class are created rather than just over-sampling with replacement. Some operations such as rotation, flipping, skew, ... have been used as natural ways in image processing to perturb the training data [32]. However, in the SMOTE technique, data are generated in a less application-specific manner and in the *feature space* rather than in the *data space*. In fact, the k nearest neighbors (originally $k = 5$) of each minority class sample is found and new synthetic samples are generated by interpolating between the sample and its k nearest neighbors. For instance, if a 200% over-sampling is required and the $k = 5$, then for each sample only two of the nearest neighbors are taken randomly and the new synthetic samples are generated in the direction of each by interpolation. The interpolation is done like this: take the difference between the feature vector (sample) under consideration and its nearest neighbor. Multiply this difference by a random number between 0 and 1, and add it to the feature vector under consideration.

CHAPTER 4: DEEP GENERATIVE ALGORITHMS

4.1 Introduction

Generative neural network models are powerful tools for learning the true underlying distribution of any kind of dataset in unsupervised settings, i.e., building a model which can represent the dataset. Three of the most commonly used families of generative models are Variational Autoencoder-Decoder (VAE), Generative Adversarial Networks (GAN) Probabilistic Diffusion (PD) models.

4.2 Bayes Theorem

In general the probability that two events, X and Y, *jointly* happen together is expressed by:

$$p(X \cap Y) = p(X|Y)p(Y) = p(Y|X)p(X) \tag{4.1}$$

Therefore, one can write:

$$p(X|Y) = \frac{p(Y|X)p(X)}{p(X)} \tag{4.2}$$

which is in fact the Bayes Theorem. In terms of the latent variable (or hypothesis) z and the observation x:

$$p(z|x) = \frac{p(x|z)p(z)}{p(x)} \tag{4.3}$$

Bayes theorem is a way to get an update or a better distribution when an observation is made [57].

Through the assumption that data have been originally generated by a much lower-dimension latent variable space (Z), Autoencoder-Decoder (AE) models learn the distribution of the latent space and map from Z (latent space) to X (real data space) [18]. Assume that there is a vec-

Symbol	Description
z	Latent variable (hypothesis)
x	Evidence, observation or data
$p(x)$	Data probability or distribution
$p(z)$	Prior distribution (latent variable or hypothesis)
$p(z\|x)$	Posterior probability
$p(x\|z)$	Likelihood of data probability

Table 4.1: Bayesian Statistics Glossary

tor of latent variable z from high dimensional space $\mathcal{Z}$, which can be sampled easily with some probability density function (PDF) $P(z)$ defined over $\mathcal{Z}$. Also, we have a series of parameterized deterministic function $X = f(z;\theta)$, with the parameter vector θ in Θ, with $f : \mathcal{Z} \times \Theta \rightarrow \mathcal{X}$. f by itself is deterministic, however, since z is random and θ is fixed, then the generated data using $X = f(z;\theta)$ is a random variable in the same space as real observations $X \in \mathcal{X}$. The parameter vector θ is to be optimized (using Maximum Likelihood method) such that we can sample z from $P(z)$ and $f(z;\theta)$ produces an X similar to the elements in our dataset (space $\mathcal{X}$) with a very high probability. However, using the observations data, we can have a better and improved distribution of the latent variables, i.e., the *posterior* $P(z|x)$, and sampling from it generates better data via $X = f(z;\theta), z \in P(z|x)$.

To find the posterior distribution Eq. 4.3 can be used. However, $p(x) = \int p(x|z)p(z)dz$ is computationally intractable. Therefore, we can approximate $p(x|z)$ by $q(x|z)$ and try to minimize the distance between the two, e.g., the *Kulback-Leibler Divergence* between them:

$$\min \ KL\left(q(x|z) \,\|\, p(x|z)\right) \tag{4.4}$$

Kulback-Leibler divergence in fact is the expectation of the information difference between the the two distributions. Information content (I) is inversely proportional to the probability of an event:

$$I_p(x) = -\log p(x) \tag{4.5}$$

$$I_q(x) = -\log q(x) \tag{4.6}$$

$$\Delta I = I_p - I_q = -\log p(x) + \log q(x) = \log\left(\frac{q(x)}{p(x)}\right) \tag{4.7}$$

and the *Kulback-Leibler Divergence* is defined as the expectation of the above difference, for example with respect to $q(x)$:

$$KL\left(q(x|z)\,||\,p(x|z)\right) = E_q[\Delta I] = \int (\Delta I)\,q(x)dx = \int q(x)\log\left(\frac{q(x)}{p(x)}\right)dx \tag{4.8}$$

or with respect to $p(x)$:

$$KL\left(p(x|z)\,||\,q(x|z)\right) = E_p[\Delta I] = \int (\Delta I)\,p(x)dx = \int p(x)\log\left(\frac{p(x)}{q(x)}\right)dx \tag{4.9}$$

Note that in general:

$$KL\left(p(x|z)\,||\,q(x|z)\right) \neq KL\left(q(x|z)\,||\,p(x|z)\right) \tag{4.10}$$

Hence the Kullback-Leibler is called a *divergence* and not a *metric* as metrics must be symmetric.

Also note that KL divergence is always non-negative.

4.3 Variational Autoencoder

The real data or observations or evidences are fed to the *encoder* and the posterior distribution of the latent variables are generated (recall $z \in \mathcal{N}(0,1)$, while the improved latent variables $z \in q_\theta(z|x)$). The decoder uses the improved latent variables and generates data belonging to the data space $\mathcal{X}$.

$$\log p(x_i) = KL\left(q_\theta(z|x_i) \,\|\, p(z)\right) + \mathbb{E}_{q_\theta(z|x_i)}\left[\log p_\phi\left(x_i|z\right)\right] \tag{4.11}$$

or:

$$\log p(x_i) = KL\left(q_\theta(z|x_i) \,\|\, p(z)\right) + \sum_z q_\theta\left(z|x\right) \log \frac{p_\phi\left(x_i|z\right)}{q_\theta\left(z|x\right)} \tag{4.12}$$

The right hand side of the above equation is called *Variational Lower Bound* of the evidences. Therefore, since $\log p(x_i)$ is a constant (distribution of the real data from the dataset), instead of minimizing $KL\left(q_\theta(z|x_i) \,\|\, p(z)\right)$, its lower bound $\mathbb{E}_{q_\theta(z|x_i)}\left[\log p_\phi\left(x_i|z\right)\right]$ can be equivalently maximized.

4.4 GAN

Generative Adversarial Network (GAN) models are inherently two-player zero-sum minimax games. Two-player games refer to games in which two participants, typically referred to as players, interact with each other in a competitive or cooperative manner. Two-player games can have different characteristics, such as being turn-based or simultaneous, zero-sum or non-zero-sum, perfect information or imperfect information. In a zero-sum game, the gain of one player is balanced by the loss of the other player. The total utility or payoff in the game remains constant, and one player's success is directly correlated with the other player's failure [5].

The two players in a GAN model are the *generator* and the *discriminator*. They both optimize the same loss function (Eq. 4.13); the *generator* tries to minimize and the *discriminator* tries to maximize the loss function.

$$\min_G \max_D V(D, G) = \mathbb{E}_{x \sim p_{data}(x)}\left[\log D\left(x\right)\right] + \mathbb{E}_{z \sim p_z(z)}\left[1 - \log\left(D\left(G\left(z\right)\right)\right)\right] \tag{4.13}$$

Note that in Eq. 4.13, unlike the VAE loss function, Eq. 4.4, there is no explicit *distribution matching* and as long as the averages, i.e., the expected value of the $\log D\left(x\right)$ and $\left(D\left(G\left(z\right)\right)\right)$ meet

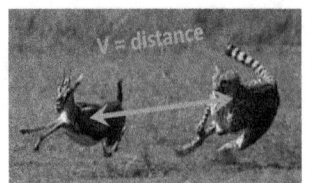

Figure 4.1: Adversarial Training

hereas, in Eq. 4.4, the optimization forces the training to match the two distributions. This is the reason that GAN models show less *diversity* compared to VAE models, i.e., not all the modalities in the real dataset are always covered in GAN models, unlike VAE models.

The two optimizations in Eq. 4.13 are done in practice sequentially. In fact for each parameter optimization for the discriminator, the parameters in the generator are updated 5 times [29]. Experience has shown that GAN models show better *fidelity* in the generated data relative to the real data than VAE models do.

4.5 WGAN

Wasserstein GAN models improve the convergence challenge in GAN models by incorporating the *Wasserstein Distance* or the *Earth Movers'* distance in their loss function.

$$W_1(p_r, p_g) = \sup_{\|f\|_L \leq 1} \mathbb{E}_{x \sim p_r}[f(x)] - \mathbb{E}_{x \sim p_g}[f(x)] \tag{4.14}$$

The Wasserstein distance measures the dissimilarity between two probability distributions by quantifying the minimum cost of transforming one distribution into the other [6]. It provides a meaningful metric for evaluating the similarity between the generated distribution and the real data distribution.

By incorporating the Wasserstein distance metric into the loss function, some of the limitations of traditional GANs are addressed:

- training instability
- mode collapse
- more stable optimization process

Instead of the original GAN objective function that uses the *Jensen-Shannon Divergence* or *Kullback-Leibler Divergence*, WGANs use a different objective function based on the Wasserstein distance. The discriminator in a WGAN is referred to as a critic, and its goal is to estimate the Wasserstein distance.

To enforce *Lipschitz continuity* in the WGAN discriminator, *weight clipping* is applied, i.e., the magnitudes of all the trainable parameters are kept bounded. It restricts the magnitude of the critic's weights within a predefined range of $[-c, c]$. However, weight clipping can lead to suboptimal performance and other issues, such as gradient vanishing or exploding. Hence, an alternative to weight clipping, called *gradient penalty*, has been proposed in later variants of WGANs, such as **WGAN-GP** (next section).

Traditional GANs often suffer from training instability, where the discriminator and generator reach an equilibrium that leads to *mode collapse* or suboptimal performance. WGANs address this issue by providing a more stable optimization process through the use of the Wasserstein distance. The continuous and meaningful nature of the Wasserstein distance allows for better gradient information, leading to more reliable and stable training.

$$\min_{G} \max_{D} V(D,G) = \min_{G} \max_{\|f\|_L \leq 1} \mathbb{E}_{x \sim p_r}[\log D(x)] - \mathbb{E}_{x \sim p_g}[D(G(z))] \quad (4.15)$$

WGAN, in general, has less sensitivity to the model architecture and also to the choice of hyperparameter in addition to the prevention of mode collapse [6].

4.6 WGAN-GP

An alternative technique for k-Lipschitz continuity constraint is *keeping the norm of the gradient always below 1*. In practice this condition (*constraint*) replaces the parameter clipping in the *soft* implementation. Using the *Lagrange* multipliers method, the constraint is used to penalize the WGAN loss function, Eq. 4.14, however, only at some random samples $\hat{x} \sim p_{\hat{x}}$ and not at every single point.

4.7 Advantages and Issues of GAN Models

GAN models, in general, have many advantages that have made the a revolutionary model in deep learning [51], among which one can refer to:

- GANs do not inherently require Markov chains because they do not rely on sequential dependencies. Instead, GANs learn to capture the *underlying distribution* of the training data and generate samples from that distribution. They can generate samples in a single step, *without the need for explicit modeling of sequential dependencies*. GANs excel at generating realistic and high-quality samples across various domains, such as images, music, and text.

- In GAN models, the training process is advantageous because it only requires backpropagation to obtain gradients and, unlike traditional Markov Chain models, doesn't involve complex inference procedures (here inference refers to making predictions or estimating values based on available information).

In an unconditional GAN model, there is no control on the modality of the data being generated [51]. However, by conditioning the model on the category of data, it is possible to direct the data generation process and generated data of some certain modality.

On the other hand, it is very challenging to scale GAN models to extremely large number (hundreds, thousands or even millions) of predicted output categories. Another issue with with

GAN models is that most of the researches so far have focuses on learning on-to-one mapping tasks between the input space and the output space. However, many real life events are of one-to-many mapping, such as, in image labeling there may be many labels that could appropriately tagged to a given image. In other words, different annotators can use different (but typically synonymous or related somehow) terms to describe the image.

One way to to address the first issue is to leverage additional information from other modalities. For instance, a vector representation of labels is learned in which geometric relations are also semantically meaningful. The key idea here is that labels should have vectors that are close to the vectors of related words, indicating their semantic similarity. Additionally, similar labels should have vectors that are mathematically close to each other in the vector space, indicating their semantic similarity, In other words, symantic similarity should indicate mathematical similarity and vice verse. In this way, geometric operations like vector addition or subtraction can be meaningful in this space. For example, subtracting the vector of "good" from the vector of "excellent" should yield a vector that represents the meaning of "very good."

On e way to address the second issue, is to use *conditional* probabilistic generative model: the input is taken to be the conditioning variable and the one-to-many mapping is instantiated as a conditional predictive distribution [51].

4.8 Conditional GAN

Regular GAN models 4.13 can be extended to *conditional GAN* models if both the generator and discriminator are conditioned on some extra information y, the *auxiliary information*, which can be either the class of the data or some information from other modalities. Foe instance, when training a GAN model for generating of dog images, the auxiliary information can be a text describing a dog, or an audio file from dog, ... This is usually referred to as *multimodal learning*. Usually, the auxiliary information is fed to the generator and discriminator as an extra layer of input [51]. The objective of a conditional GAN looks like the following:

$$\min_{G} \max_{D} V(D,G) = \mathbb{E}_{x \sim p_{data}(x)} \left[\log D\left(x|y\right) \right] + \mathbb{E}_{z \sim p_z(z)} \left[1 - \log \left(D\left(G\left(z|y\right) \right) \right) \right] \quad (4.16)$$

4.9 Denoising Diffusion Probabilistic Models

Denoising Diffusion Probabilistic Models (DDPM), similar to the VAE model, are *variational-based model* [56] where the objective is to find the distribution of the dataset explicitly [45]. There are two processes in a DDPM: *forward process* and *backward process*. In the forward process, q, noise is added gradually to a datapoint $x_0 \sim q(x_0)$. The generated noisy samples are x_1 through x_T, which are in fact the latent variables of the variational model. The added noise is a Gaussian noise which is added at each step according to a variance schedule given by β_t [38]:

$$q(x_t|x_{t-1}) = \mathcal{N}\left(x_t; \sqrt{1-\beta_t}x_t, \beta_t \boldsymbol{I}\right) \quad (4.17)$$

Defining $\alpha_t = 1 - \beta_t$ and $\bar{\alpha}_t = \prod_{s=0}^{t} \alpha_s$, $q(x_t|x_0)$ can be expressed in a closed form:

$$\begin{aligned} q(x_t|x_0) &= \mathcal{N}\left(x_t; \sqrt{\bar{\alpha}_t}\, x_0, (1-\bar{\alpha}_t)\, \boldsymbol{I}\right) \\ &= \sqrt{\bar{\alpha}_t}\, x_0 + \epsilon\sqrt{1-\bar{\alpha}_t}, \quad \epsilon \sim \mathcal{N}(0, \boldsymbol{I}) \end{aligned} \quad (4.18)$$

where, $1 - \bar{\alpha}_t$ is the variance of the noise at any arbitrary step and can be used directly, instead of β_t. Using Bayes theorem, it can be proved that the posterior of the reverse process $q(x_{t-1}|x_t, x_0)$ is also a Gaussian distribution [38]:

$$q(x_{t-1}|x_t, x_0) = \mathcal{N}\left(x_{t-1}; \tilde{\mu}_t\left(x_t, x_0\right), \tilde{\beta}_t \boldsymbol{I}\right) \quad (4.19)$$

with:

$$\begin{cases} \tilde{\mu}_t(x_t, x_0) = \frac{\sqrt{\bar{\alpha}_{t-1}} \beta_t}{1-\bar{\alpha}_t} x_0 + \frac{\sqrt{\alpha_t}(1-\bar{\alpha}_{t-1})}{1-\bar{\alpha}_t} \\ \tilde{\beta}_t = \frac{1-\bar{\alpha}_{t-1}}{1-\bar{\alpha}_t} \beta_t \end{cases} \quad (4.20)$$

To sample from $q(x_0)$, knowing $q(x_{t-1}|x_t)$, we can start from $q(x_T)$ and then sample the reverse steps $q(x_{t-1}|x_t)$ till we reach x_0. Under certain assumptions on β_t and T, sampling x_T is trivial so pure noise is usually used. However, since $q(x_{t-1}|x_t)$ is *intractable*, a neural network is trained to approximate it. Also since $\beta_t \to 0$ and $q(x_{t-1}|x_t)$ approaches a diagonal Gaussian distribution, as $T \to \infty$, it would be sufficient to train a neural network to predict the mean μ_θ and the diagonal covariance Σ_θ:

$$p_\theta(x_{t-1}|x_t) = \mathcal{N}(x_{t-1}; \mu_\theta(x_t, t), \Sigma_\theta(x_t, t)) \quad (4.21)$$

The variational lower-bound loss function of L_{vlb} for $p_\theta(x_0)$ is:

$$L_{vlb} = L_0 + L_1 + \cdots + L_{T-1} + L_T \quad (4.22)$$

$$L_0 = -\log p_\theta(x_0|x_1) \quad (4.23)$$

$$L_{t-1} = D_{KL}(q(x_{t-1}|x_t, x_0) \parallel p_\theta(x_{t-1}|x_t)) \quad (4.24)$$

$$L_T - D_{KL}(q(x_T|x_0) \parallel p(x_T)) \quad (4.25)$$

Ho *et al.* [38] used a simplified loss function in which a neural network $\epsilon_\theta(x_t, t)$ is trained to to predict ϵ from Eq. 4.18:

$$L_{simple} = E_{t \sim [1,T], x_0 \sim q(x_0), \epsilon \sim \mathcal{N}(0,I)} \left[\|\epsilon - \epsilon_\theta(x_t, t)\|^2 \right] \quad (4.26)$$

Then $\mu_\theta(x_t, t)$ can be derived from $\epsilon_\theta(x_t, t)$:

$$\mu_\theta(x_t, t) = \frac{1}{\sqrt{\alpha_t}} \left(x_t - \frac{1-\alpha_t}{\sqrt{1-\bar{\alpha}_t}} \epsilon_\theta(x_t, t) \right) \quad (4.27)$$

L_{simple} does not provide any signal for training $\Sigma_\theta(x_t, t)$. So, instead of learning $\Sigma_\theta(x_t, t)$, it is fixed to a constant, i.e.,: $\Sigma_\theta(x_t, t) = \sigma_t^2 I$ where $\sigma_t^2 = \beta_t$ or $\sigma_t^2 = \tilde{\beta}_t = \frac{1-\bar{\alpha}_{t-1}}{1-\bar{\alpha}_t}\beta_t$ which are the upper and lower bounds for the true reverse process' step variance, respectively.

4.10 Improved DDPM

Log-likelihood is a metric in generative modeling and is an indication of the coverage of the existing modes in the dataset by the model [62]. Also, it has been shown that it has a great impact on the quality of samples and learnt feature representations [36]. Nichol *et al.* [56] made a few modification on the DDPM developed by Ho *et al.* [38] to achieve better Log-likelihood, which are introduced below very briefly.

4.10.1 Learned Sigma

$\Sigma_\theta(x_t, t)$ is the variance of the reverse process. Nichol *et al.* [56] argue that by increasing the number of the diffusion steps, the role of the mean $\mu_\theta(x_t, t)$ becomes more dominant than variance $\Sigma_\theta(x_t, t)$ in determining the *distribution* of the data. They also argue that not fixing, rather learning the variance $\Sigma_\theta(x_t, t)$ would provide a better choice and the Log-likelihood is improved. They suggested an interpolation between β and $\tilde{\beta}$ (the two extremes of the lower and the higher bounds) for the parameterization of the variance. In fact, their model outputs a vector v which interpolates between the two fixed extreme values (β and $\tilde{\beta}$) and has the same dimension as the data:

$$\Sigma_\theta(x_t, t) = \exp\left(v \log \beta_t + (1-v) \log \tilde{\beta}_t\right) \tag{4.28}$$

Since L_{simple} (Eq. 4.26) is independent of $\Sigma_\theta(x_t, t)$, they suggested a new hybrid objective to learn $\Sigma_\theta(x_t, t)$:

$$L_{hybrid} = L_{simple} + \lambda L_{vlb} \tag{4.29}$$

in which λ is set to a low value of 0.001 to prevent L_{vlb} from overwhelming L_{simple}.

4.10.2 Noise Schedule

Linear noising was used in the original DDPM by Ho *et al.* [38], which Nichol *et al.* [56] found sub-optimal for lower resolution (i.e. 64×64 or 32×32) image processing. Instead, they proposed a *cosine* schedule, which retain information in the noisy images longer in the noising process steps, as opposed to the strong *linear* schedule in which the noisy images become pure noise much earlier in the steps and the information in the image is destroyed much more quickly in the noising (Fig. 4.2 and 4.3):

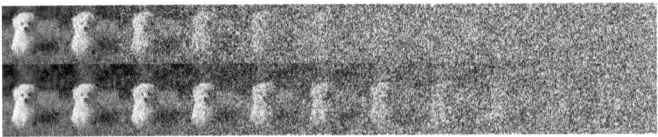

Figure 4.2: DDPM with *Linear* (top) and *Cosine* (bottom) Noise Schedules

As seen, the latents in the last quarter of *Linear* schedule are pure noise whereas *Cosine* schedule adds noise more slowly [56].

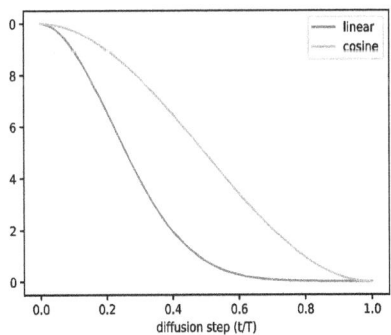

Figure 4.3: Variation of $\bar{\alpha}_t$ with time steps in *linear* and *cosine* schedules

The propsed *cosine* noising schedule is defined where $\bar{\alpha}_t$ is:

$$\bar{\alpha}_t = \frac{f(t)}{f(0)} \quad , \quad f(t) = \cos\left(\frac{t/T + s}{1 + s} \cdot \frac{\pi}{2}\right)^2 \tag{4.30}$$

with s being an offset parameter set at $s = 0.008$. The offset s is to prevent β_t from being too small near $t = 0$, since having even tiny amounts of noise can make the prediction of ϵ hard for the network. So s is chosen such that $\sqrt{\beta_0}$ is slightly smaller than the pixel bin size $\frac{1}{127.5}$ which produces $s = 0.008$.

It should be noted that $\beta_t = 1 - \frac{\bar{\alpha}_t}{\bar{\alpha}_{t-1}}$. In practice, β_t is clipped to be always less than 0.999 to prevent any singularities at the end of the diffusion process near $t = T$. The *cosine* schedule is designed to have a linear drop-off of $\bar{\alpha}_t$ in the middle of the process, while changing very little near the extremes of $t = 0$ and $t = T$ to prevent abrupt changes in noise level. Fig. 4.2 shows how $\bar{\alpha}_t$ progresses for both schedules. We can see that the linear schedule from Ho *et al.* [38] falls towards zero much faster, destroying information more quickly than necessary.

4.10.3 Importance-sampled L_{vlb}

Nichol *et al.* [56] found that, contrary to their expectation, optimizing L_{hybrid} achieves better log-likelihood rather than optimizing L_{vlb} directly, which they believe was caused by L_{vlb} and its gradient being more *noisy*. It was confirmed by evaluating *gradient noise scale* [50] for models trained with both objectives. Therefore, the variance of L_{vlb} should be reduced to in order to be optimized directly. It was found that sampling t uniformly causes unnecessary noise in L_{vlb} objective function. So, in order to reduce the variance of L_{vlb}, they employed *importance sampling* rather than sampling uniformly throughout the samples:

$$L_{vlb} = \mathbb{E}_{t \sim p_t}\left[\frac{L_t}{p_t}\right], \quad \text{where} \quad p_t \propto \sqrt{\mathbb{E}\left[L_t^2\right]} \quad \text{and} \quad \sum p_t = 1 \quad (4.31)$$

in which they kept a 10-step history for the evaluation of $\mathbb{E}\left[L_t^2\right]$ which is updated dynamically. At the beginning of training, t is sample uniformly till 10 samples are drawn for every $t \in [0, T-1]$. Using importance sampling they could achieve their best log-likelihoods with considerably less noisy objective than the uniformly sampled objective. The experience also confirmed that the objective L_{vlb} becomes much less noisy. However, importance sampling technique does not make any improvement on the less noisy L_{hybrid} objective [56].

CHAPTER 5: EVALUATION METRICS

5.1 Introduction

Evaluation Metrics assess the performance and effectiveness of machine learning models, so that models can be discriminated from each other based on the value generated by the evaluation metrics [43]. They provide objective criteria to measure how well models are functioning.

Discriminative models and *Generative* models are the two of the most commonly used models in deep learning.

5.2 Discriminative Models

Discriminative models focus on learning the *boundary* or *decision boundary* between different classes or categories in the data [43]. Their primary goal is to *discriminate* or *classify* the input data into predefined classes. These models learn the conditional probability distribution of the output given the input data. In other words, they directly model the mapping from input features to output labels.

Popular examples of discriminative models include logistic regression, support vector machines (SVMs), and most variants of neural networks used for *classification* tasks. Discriminative models are often preferred when the primary interest lies in classification or predicting the label of new instances based on the available features.

The evaluation metrics used in discriminative models are designed measure how well the *discrimination* or *classification* between various classes of data has been made. The common evaluation metrics in this category of models are: Overall Accuracy, Precision, Recall and F1-Score, Confusion Matrix, AUC-ROC and AUC-PR.

5.3 Generative Models

Generative models, on the other hand, aim to learn the *underlying probability distribution of the data* [11, 13]. Instead of focusing solely on classifying data points, generative models try to generate new samples that resemble the original data distribution. These models learn the *joint probability distribution* of the input features and the output labels.

Generative models can be used to generate new samples from the learned distribution or to estimate the probability of a particular input data point. They capture the underlying patterns and structure of the data, allowing for the synthesis of new instances that resemble the training data.

Popular examples of generative models include Gaussian Mixture Models (GMMs), Hidden Markov Models (HMMs), Variational Autoencoders (VAEs), and Generative Adversarial Networks (GANs).

Evaluation metrics for generative models are different from discriminative models, as they should focus on assessing the quality of generated samples and the model's ability to capture the data distribution. Some commonly used metrics include:

Log-Likelihood: It measures how well the generative model approximates the true data distribution. A lower log-likelihood indicates a better model fit to the training data.

Perplexity: This metric provides an alternative interpretation of the log-likelihood. It quantifies how well a generative model predicts a held-out or test set of data. Lower perplexity values indicate better model performance.

Inception Score: Primarily used for evaluating generative models in image synthesis tasks, the Inception Score measures the quality and diversity of generated images. It leverages an Inception classifier to evaluate the generated samples based on their class probabilities and evaluates the diversity through the entropy of these probabilities.

Fréchet Inception Distance (FID): Another popular metric for image synthesis, FID compares the generated samples with the real data distribution by computing the Frã©chet distance between their feature representations extracted from a pre-trained Inception network. Lower FID scores indicate better quality and similarity to the real data distribution.

It's worth noting that these metrics represent a subset of the evaluation methods available for discriminative and generative models. Depending on the specific task and domain, other metrics may be more appropriate or additional metrics may be developed to evaluate the performance of deep learning models.

5.4 Some Basic Concepts Used in Evaluation Metrics

There are some concepts that are used in definition of evaluation metrics [43]:

- *Negative Class:* The *Negative* class usually represent the *status quo* (prevalent or Normal case)

- *Positive Class:* Any *change* or abnormality relative to the Negative class is considered as the *Positive*

- *True Positive:* The data belongs to the *Positive* class and model predicts it as *Positive*

- *True Negative:* The data belongs to the *Negative* class and model predicts it as *Negative*

- *False Positive:* The data belongs to the *Negative* class but the model predicts it as *Positive*

- *False Negative:* The data belongs to the *Positive* class but the model predicts it as *Negative*

5.5 Evaluation Metrics for Discriminative Models

5.5.1 Confusion Matrix

Confusion Matrix is an square matrix with the number of rows and columns equal to the number of classes. The vertical axis represents the *predicted classes* while the vertical axis represents the *actual classes*. The elements on the main diagonal signifies the number of **True Positives** expressed in percentages (frequencies) or counts. The off-diagonal elements of the matrix show the counts/frequencies of incorrectly classified elements (above and below the main diagonal values represent *False Positives* and the *False Negatives*, respectively. Confusion Matrix is extremely useful for measuring precision-recall, Specificity, Accuracy, and most importantly, AUC-ROC curves.

performance of classification at a glance

Vertical axis: **Predicted** classes
Horizontal axis: **Actual** classes

Number of predictions in each cell
# of class A predicted as class A
# of class A predicted as class B
# of class A predicted as class C
...

Sum of CM must be dataset support

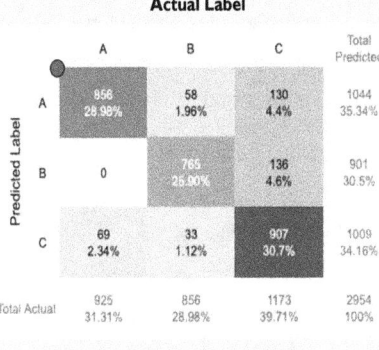

Figure 5.2: Confusion Matrix - Multiclass

5.5.2 Overall Accuracy

Overall Accuracy is defined as the fraction of all predictions that are correct:

$$Overall\ Accuracy = \frac{Correct\ Predictions}{Total\ Predictions} = \frac{TP + TN}{TP + TN + FP + FN} \quad (5.1)$$

Overall Accuracy is not a good metrics, especially in class-imbalanced dataset. Because, for instance assume that there are only 5% of a test set is *Positive* and we have a very poor classifier whose output is fixed at *Positive*, i.e., 100% of the times, the prediction is *Positive*. Therefore, this classifier's *Overall Accuracy* is 95%, which we already know is a very poor classifier.

5.5.3 Precision

Precision measures the proportion of correctly predicted positive instances out of all instances predicted as positive. Precision provides insights into the model's ability to avoid false positives, that is, correctly identifying positive instances while minimizing the misclassification of negative instances as positives. A high precision score indicates a low rate of false positives and a more reliable positive prediction by the model.

$$Precision = \frac{TP}{all\ P} = \frac{TP}{TP+FP} = \frac{1}{1+\frac{FP}{TP}} \qquad (5.2)$$

As TP is always to be maximized, *Precision* is used when FP is to be minimized, i.e., when the model is avoid False Positives.

5.5.4 Recall or Sensitivity

The *Recall* score, also known as sensitivity or true positive rate (TPR), is a metric used to evaluate the performance of a classification model, particularly in scenarios where the detection of positive instances is of higher importance.

Recall measures the proportion of actual positive instances that are correctly identified as positive by the model. It is used when FN is to be minimized and to avoid *False Negatives*. It answers the question: *Of all the positive instances in the dataset, how many did the model correctly identify?*

$$Recall = \frac{TP}{TP+FN} = \frac{1}{1+\frac{FN}{TP}} \qquad (5.3)$$

5.5.5 F1-Score

F1-Score combines Precision and Recall scores and used when both FP and FN are equally important and neither should be avoided. *F1-Score* is in fact a harmonic average of *Precision* and *Recall*:

$$\frac{1}{F1} = \frac{1}{2}\left(\frac{1}{Precision} + \frac{1}{Recall}\right) \qquad (5.4)$$

$$F1 = 2 \cdot \frac{Precision \times Recall}{Precision + Recall} \qquad (5.5)$$

5.5.6 AUC-ROC

AUC ROC (Area Under the Receiver Operating Characteristic Curve) is a widely used evaluation metric in machine learning to measure the performance of binary classification models. It provides a single scalar value that represents the overall quality of the model's predictions.

AUC ROC is applicable primarily to *binary classification* problems where the task is to classify data into one of two classes, referred to as *positive* and *negative* classes. Examples include classifying emails as spam or not spam, determining whether a customer will churn or not, or predicting whether a patient has a particular disease.

Receiver Operating Characteristic (ROC) Curve is a graphical representation of the performance of a binary classifier. It is created by plotting the true positive rate (TPR) against the false positive rate (FPR) at various classification thresholds. The TPR, also known as *sensitivity* or *recall*, represents the proportion of positive instances correctly classified as positive, while the FPR represents the proportion of negative instances incorrectly classified as positive. Each point on the ROC curve corresponds to a particular threshold setting.

AUC ROC represents the area under the ROC curve. It quantifies the overall performance of the classifier across all possible threshold settings. The *AUC ROC* value ranges from 0 to 1, where a higher value indicates better classification performance. An *AUC ROC* of 1 indicates a perfect classifier, while an *AUC ROC* of 0.5 suggests a random classifier that performs no better than chance. Figure 5.3 shows a sample of AUC ROC plot (https://www.researchgate.net/figure/An-example-of-ROC-curves-with-good-AUC-09-and-satisfactory-AUC-065-parameters_fig2_276079439).

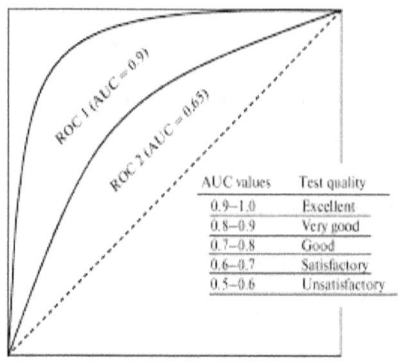

Figure 5.3: AUC ROC

The interpretation of *AUC ROC* is as follows:

- AUC = 1: The model has perfect discrimination power, meaning it can perfectly separate the positive and negative instances

- AUC > 0.5: The model performs better than random guessing. The higher the AUC, the better the model's ability to distinguish between the positive and negative classes

- AUC = 0.5: The model has no discrimination power and performs as good as random guessing

- AUC < 0.5: The model performs worse than random guessing, suggesting that its predictions are inverted or incorrect

AUC ROC is commonly used because it is *insensitive to the imbalanced nature of the dataset*, meaning it can handle cases where the number of positive and negative instances differs significantly. It also provides a single metric that is easy to interpret and compare across different models.

Multi-class AUC ROC

multiclass AUC ROC provides a comprehensive evaluation of a multiclass classification model's performance by extending the binary AUC ROC to handle multiple classes using the one-vs-all strategy. It is a useful metric to assess how well a model can discriminate between different classes and make confident predictions.

In multiclass classification, one common approach is the *one-vs-rest* (also known as *one-vs-all*) strategy. This approach trains multiple binary classifiers, where each classifier distinguishes one class from the rest of the classes. For example, if you have 5 classes (A, B, C, D, E), you would train five binary classifiers: A vs. rest, B vs. rest, C vs. rest, D vs. rest, and E vs. rest. During inference, the class with the highest predicted probability across all binary classifiers is assigned as the final predicted class.

To calculate the multiclass AUC-ROC, we need to aggregate the binary AUC-ROC scores obtained from each one-vs-rest classifier. The AUC-ROC for each binary classifier represents the ability of the model to distinguish between the positive class and the rest of the classes. The multiclass AUC-ROC can be computed using different averaging strategies, such as *micro-average*, *macro-average*, or *weighted average*:

- ***Micro-Average:*** In the micro-average approach, we compute the TPR and FPR globally across all classes. We concatenate the true positive, false positive, true negative, and false negative counts from all classes and calculate the TPR and FPR. Then, we compute the AUC-ROC from the combined TPR and FPR values.

- ***Macro-Average:*** In the macro-average approach, we calculate the AUC-ROC for each class separately. Then, we average the AUC-ROC scores obtained from all classes to obtain the final multiclass AUC-ROC score. This approach gives equal weight to each class, regardless of the class-imbalance.

- ***Weighted Average:*** The weighted average approach is similar to the macro-average approach, but it takes into account the class-imbalance. Each class's AUC-ROC score is weighted by the proportion of samples belonging to that class. This means that the AUC-ROC of larger classes contributes more to the final multiclass AUC-ROC score.

It's worth mentioning that there is also another multiclass strategy called *one-vs-one*, where we create binary classifiers for each possible pair of classes. The concept remains similar to *One-vs-all*, but it requires $\frac{C \times (C-1)}{2}$ (C: number of classes) classifiers, which can be computationally expensive for large C. The *One-vs-all* strategy is often preferred due to its simplicity and scalability.

5.5.7 AUC-PR

the Area Under the Precision-Recall Curve (AUC PR) metric is a valuable tool for assessing the performance of classification models, especially in scenarios with imbalanced datasets or when the focus is on positive instances. It quantifies the trade-off between precision and recall, providing a comprehensive measure of the model's ability to identify positive instances accurately while minimizing false positives.

AUC PR is the area under the Precision-Recall curve. The AUC PR value summarizes the model's performance across all possible thresholds, providing an aggregate measure of the model's ability to balance precision and recall. A perfect AUC PR score would be 1.0, indicating a model with perfect precision and recall at all thresholds. This means the model can perfectly distinguish positive and negative instances. An AUC PR score of 0.0 would mean that the model's predictions are no better than random guessing. Figure 5.4 and 5.5 show some samples of AUC PR plots (https://towardsai.net/p/l/precision-recall-curve).

AUC PR is particularly useful when dealing with imbalanced datasets, where the number of negative instances far exceeds the number of positive instances. It gives insights into how well a model can identify positive instances while maintaining a low number of false positives. A higher AUC PR score indicates better model performance, reflecting a better trade-off between precision and recall.

The AUC PR is sensitive to the imbalance of the classes, so it provides a more reliable evaluation for imbalanced datasets compared to metrics like accuracy.

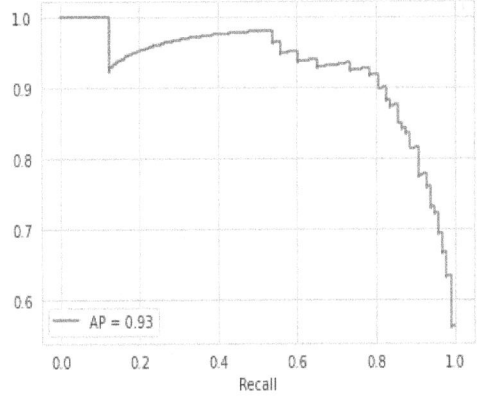

Figure 5.4: AUC PR - Monoclass

Figure 5.5: AUC PR - Multiclass

5.6 Evaluation Metrics for Generative Models

5.6.1 Background

Given a set of real data $\{X_i\}$ with the distribution of $P(X)$ and a set of generated data $\{Y_j\}$ generated by a generative model Q, i.e., with a distribution $Q(Y)$, it is assumed that we can freely sample from both sets. We need an algorithm to assess how likely the sets of samples are arising from the same distribution [55]. If the above distributions are tractable, statistical distant measures (such as *Kullback-Leibler Divergence* or *Expected Likelihood*) can be used, otherwise, when $P(X)$ is complex, high-dimensional as in real images or otherwise, it becomes difficult to apply these measures naively [71]. That's why, the evaluation generative models and the samples from them are still among the hot and actively researched topics.

5.6.2 Evaluation Pipeline

The evaluation metrics for image generative models largely follow the following stages:

- ***Embedding:*** Embed real $\{X_i\}$ and fake $\{Y_j\}$ data into a Euclidean space $\mathbb{R}^D$ through a non-linear mapping f like CNN feature extractors

- **Build Feature Space:** Construct real and fake distributions over the feature space $\mathbb{R}^D$ with the embedded samples $\{f(X_i)\}$ and $\{f(Y_j)\}$

- **Compare Distributions:** Quantify the discrepancy between the two distributions

Embedding

When the data are high-dimensional, it is very hard to define a sensible distant measure over the input space. For instance, the *Euclidean* distance, i.e., the L_2 norm $\|X_i - Y_j\|$, is not a proper metric, because two identical inputs will show a huge distance if they are shifted relative to each other even by one pixel (one-pixel translation) [71].

In order to address this issue, the ImageNet pre-trained CNN feature extractor has been developed and used as the embedding function f to map the high-dimensional input data into a simpler feature space ([37, 46, 66, 67] base on the reasoning that the L_2 norm in the feature space $\|f(X_i) - f(Y_j)\|$ predicts sensible proxies closer to human perceptual metrics.

Feature Space and Comparing the Distributions

- **Non-Parametric Approach:** Bengio et al. [8] introduced *Parzen Window Estimates* to approximate the likelihoods of fake samples Y_j by estimating the density $P(X)$ with Gaussian kernels around the real samples X_i.

- **Parametric Approach:** The *Inception Score* (IS) and the *Fréchet Inception Score* (FID) are two parametric evaluation metrics used to assess the quality and diversity of generated images. The Inception Score, introduced by Salimans et al. [67], is based on the idea that a good generator should produce diverse images that are both visually appealing and representative of different classes. The metric utilizes a pre-trained Inception neural network, which is a CNN designed for image classification. To calculate the Inception Score, the generator produces a set of generated images, and each image is passed through the Inception network to obtain a probability distribution over classes. The scores are then computed by taking the average of the Kullback-Leibler (KL) divergence between the class distribution of each generated image and the overall class distribution of the generated images. Higher Inception Scores indicate better quality and diversity in the generated images.

The Fréchet Inception Score (FID), developed by Heusel *et al.* [37], measures the similarity between the two distributions based on the Freéchet distance function [19], aka the Wasserstein-2 distance. To compute the FID, the feature representations of real and generated images are extracted using an intermediate layer of the Inception network. The mean μ and the covariance Σ for $\{X\}$ and $\{Y\}$ are estimated, assuming they are Gaussians. The Fréchet distance is then calculated between these two Gausian distributions to quantify the dissimilarity. Lower FID scores indicate better similarity between the real and generated image distributions, implying higher quality and realism in the generated images. FID has been reported to generally match with human judgements [37]; it has been the most popular metric for image generative models in the last couple of years [13].

While single-value metrics like IS and FID have led interesting advances in the field by ranking generative models, they are not ideal for diagnostic purposes, because they do not capture the trade-off between fidelity and diversity of the generated data. Some two-value metrics are introduced which capture these two concepts separately [55].

5.6.3 Fidelity and Diversity

Fidelity

Fidelity refers to the extent to which the generated samples closely resemble or faithfully represent the target distribution, such as real data. A generative model with high fidelity produces outputs that are highly realistic, similar to the training data, and indistinguishable from real examples. Fidelity is often associated with qualities like image sharpness, texture details, and overall visual coherence. High fidelity indicates that the generated samples exhibit high quality and are difficult to distinguish from real data.

Diversity

Diversity refers to the variety or richness of the generated samples. A generative model with high diversity is capable of producing a wide range of distinct outputs, capturing different modes or variations present in the target distribution. Diversity is an important aspect as it ensures that the generative model does not produce repetitive or overly similar samples. High diversity indicates that the generated samples cover a broad range of possibilities, showing different styles, poses, colors, or other relevant characteristics.

Balancing fidelity and diversity is a crucial challenge in generative modeling. While high fidelity ensures realistic and accurate representations, high diversity prevents mode collapse (where the model generates limited or repetitive samples) and encourages exploration of the entire target distribution. Achieving both fidelity and diversity is a desirable goal for generative models to produce high-quality and diverse outputs.

5.6.4 Precision and Recall in Generative Models

Sajjadi *et al.* [66] have reported a pathological case where two generative models have similar FID scores, while their qualitative fidelity and diversity results are different [55]. They proposed the *precision* and *recall* metrics for generative models based on the estimated supports of the real and fake distributions.

Precision

Precision is defined as the portion of $Q(Y)$ that can be generated by $P(X)$.

Recall

recall is symmetrically defined as the portion of $P(X)$ that can be generated by $Q(Y)$.

While conceptually useful, they have multiple practical drawbacks. It assumes that the embedding space is uniformly dense, relies on the initialisation-sensitive k-means algorithm for support estimation, and produces an infinite number of values as the metric.

Naeem et al. [55] introduced the novel *Density* and *Coverage*. However, They do not claim that they have found the ultimate solution to the universal comparison metric for generative models.

5.7 Distance Functions or Similarity Measures

Distance Functions (DF) or *Similarity Measures* are mathematical functions which take two data points from the input (dataset) space and generate one single scalar output that quantifies the similarity (or dissimilarity or distance) between its two inputs.

$$\forall\ x, y \in \mathscr{R}^{(m,n)} \qquad DF(\mathbf{x}, \mathbf{y}) : \mathscr{R}^{(m,n)} \times \mathscr{R}^{m,n} \to \mathscr{R} \qquad (5.6)$$

There are numerous distance functions available, each suitable for different types of data and applications. Some common distance functions include *Euclidean distance, Manhattan distance, Cosine similarity, Jaccard similarity, Dynamic Time Warping Distance, Fréchet Distance.*

Below, some of the most important similarity metrics which are used in this study are discussed briefly.

5.7.1 Euclidean Distance

Euclidean distance is the most familiar metrics exists. Very briefly it is the square root of the sum of the squares of corresponding elements between the two data points:

$$\forall\ X, Y \in \mathscr{R}^n, X = (x_1, x_2, \ldots, x_n), Y = (y_1, y_2, \ldots, y_n)$$
$$d_{euc} = \sqrt{(x_1 - y_1)^2 + (x_2 - y_2)^2 + \cdots + (x_n - y_n)^2} \qquad (5.7)$$

In Euclidean Distance metric both the data points must be of the same dimensions. The biggest disadvantage of this metric is that if the two input data points are identical, with one of them is shifted just by one pixel, the produced output will be huge. This makes the application of Euclidean distance very limited.

5.7.2 Dynamic Time Warping (DTW)

Dynamic Time Warping (DTW) belongs to a family of measures known as *elastic dissimilarity measures* and it works by optimally aligning (warping) the time scale in a way that the accumulated cost of this alignment is minimal [10]. It is probably the most popular distance measure for time series data, because it captures flexible similarities under time distortions. It usually works on temporal sequence inputs which may vary in speed. For example, if two persons walk similarly however with different speeds, it can detect the similarity. It has been applied to temporal sequence of video, audio and graphic data. It has particularly applications in speech recognition, signature recognition and speaker recognition.

The basic idea behind DTW is to find an optimal alignment between two sequences by warping and stretching the time axis to minimize the total distance or dissimilarity. The algorithm works as follows:

- Create a matrix D with dimensions (mxn), where m and n represent the lengths of the two sequences being compared.

- Initialize the matrix with large values or infinity

- Set the starting point (0, 0) of the matrix to zero

- Calculate the pairwise distance between all elements of the sequences and fill the matrix accordingly

- Starting from the top-left corner of the matrix, find the optimal path that minimizes the total distance

- Traverse the matrix, moving either horizontally, vertically, or diagonally, and accumulate the distances

- Once the path reaches the bottom-right corner of the matrix, the accumulated distance represents the DTW distance between the two sequences

DTW has various applications in machine learning. It can be used as a distance metric in clustering algorithms, where it helps identify groups of similar time series data. It is also employed in classification tasks, where it enables the recognition of patterns or activities in temporal data. Additionally, DTW can be used in anomaly detection to identify abnormal patterns that deviate significantly from normal behavior.

It calculates the optimal match between two given sequences by constructing a *cost matrix* D based on the two time-series being compared, x and y. The elements of matrix D are defined, by a recurrent formula:

$$D_{i,j} = f(x_i, y_j) + \min\{D_{i-1,j}, D_{i,j-1}, D_{i-1,j-1}\} \tag{5.8}$$

For $i = 1, \ldots M$ and $j = 1, \ldots N$ where M and N are the lengths of the two input data points. The total cost function $f(.,.)$ also called sample dissimilarity function, is usually the Euclidean distance. The Final DTW value typically corresponds to the total accumulated cost, i.e.,:

$$d_{DTW}(x, y) = D_{M,N} \tag{5.9}$$

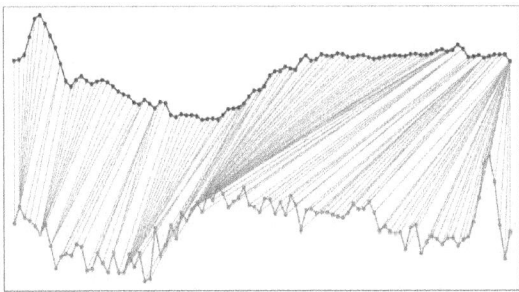

Figure 5.6: Dynamic Time Warping [87]

5.7.3 Fréchet Distance Measure

One of the major applications of C function is in the study of moving objects and comparing their trajectories (e.g., hurricane path prediction, the study of animal migrations, time series paths ...). the intuition behind the Fréchet Distance function is as follows [21]:

> A man is walking a dog on a leash: the man can move on one curve, the dog on the other; both may vary their speed, but backtracking is not allowed. What is the length of the **shortest leash** that is sufficient for traversing both curves?

If $P = \{u_1, u_2, \ldots, u_p\}$ and $Q = \{v_1, v_2, \ldots, v_q\}$ are two time series (trajectories to be compared), a **coupling L** (the leash) between P and Q is defined as the set of links. Note that the leash length cannot be tightened or extended during the traversal.

$$(u_{a_1}, v_{b_1}), (u_{a_2}, v_{b_2}), \ldots, (u_{a_m}, v_{b_m}) \qquad (5.10)$$

such that:

$$a_1 = 1, b_1 = 1, a_m = p, \text{ and } b_m = q$$

$$\forall \ i \in [1, q]:$$

$$a_{i+1} = \begin{cases} a_i \\ \text{or} \\ a_i + 1 \end{cases} \qquad b_{i+1} = \begin{cases} b_i \\ \text{or} \\ b_i + 1 \end{cases}$$

The length $\|L\|$ of the coupling L is defined as the longest (maximum Euclidean distance) in the link L:

$$\|L\| = \max_{\forall i \in [1,m]} d(u_{a_i}, v_{b_i}) \tag{5.11}$$

Then the Fréchet distance between P and Q is defined as [7]:

$$\delta_{dF} = \min\{\|L\| \mid L \text{ is a coupling between } P \text{ and } Q\} \tag{5.12}$$

The Fréchet distance is a robust metric that considers both the geometry and order of points in the curves being compared. It captures the notion of closeness in terms of how paths are traversed and can handle various types of data, including time series, trajectories, and shape representations.

5.7.4 Maximum Mean Discrepancy (MMD)

Nowadays, data are being generated at an incredible rate in wide variety of ways, in different labs with different techniques to synthetic data with various generative models. These data should be combined in order to be analyzed together. The fundamental question in integration of these data is [12]:

- *Were the two sets of samples X and Y generated by the same distribution?*

In data integration terms, are these two samples part of the same larger dataset, or should these data be treated as originating from two different sources? If the distributions are different, by integrating the sets, new modalities will be introduced. If they use identical techniques on identical subjects but obtain results that are not generated by the same distribution, then this might indicate that there is a difference in the way they generate data, and that their results should not be integrated directly.

The above fundamental question is often referred to as *two-sample* or *homogeneity* problem. Let $\mathcal{F}$ be a class of functions $f : \mathcal{X} \to \mathbb{R}$. Let p and q Borel distributions, and let $X = (x_1, \ldots, x_m)$ and $y = (y_1, \ldots, y_n)$ be samples composed of independent and identically distributed observations drawn from p and q, respectively. We define the *Maximum Mean Discrepancy* (MMD) as [12]:

$$MMD\left[\mathcal{F}, X, Y\right] := \sup_{f \in \mathcal{F}} \left(\mathbb{E}_p\left[f(x)\right] - \mathbb{E}_q\left[f(y)\right]\right) \tag{5.13}$$

and its empirical estimate as:

$$MMD[\mathcal{F}, X, Y] := \sup_{f \in \mathcal{F}} \left(\frac{1}{m} \sum_{i=1}^{m} f(x_i) - \frac{1}{n} \sum_{j=1}^{n} f(y_j) \right) \quad (5.14)$$

Intuitively, we can claim that MMD will vanish *if and only if* $p = q$. Let $\mathcal{H}$ be a complete inner product Hilbert space of functions $f : \mathcal{X} \to \mathbb{R}$. $f(x)$ can be expressed as an *inner product* through:

$$f(x) = \langle f \phi(x) \rangle_{\mathcal{H}} \quad (5.15)$$

where $\phi : \mathcal{X} \to \mathcal{H}$ is known as the *feature space map* from x to $\mathcal{H}$. The inner product of two feature maps is called *kernel*, $k(x, x') := \langle \phi(x), \phi(x') \rangle_{\mathcal{H}}$. Of particular interest are cases where we have an analytic expression for k that can be computed quickly, despite $\mathcal{H}$ being high- or even infinite dimensional. An example of an infinite-dimensional $\mathcal{H}$ is corresponding to the Gaussian kernel:

$$k(x, x') = \frac{\exp\left(-\|x - x'\|^2\right)}{2\sigma^2} \quad (5.16)$$

Theorem 1. *Let p, q be Borel probability measures on $\mathcal{X}$ a compact subset of a metric space, and let $\mathcal{H}$ be a universal reproducing kernel Hilbert space with unit ball $\mathcal{F}$. Then $MMD[\mathcal{F}, p, q] = 0$ if and only if $p = q$.*

moreover, if $\mu_p := \mathbb{E}_p[\phi(x)]$, then under these conditions, one may rewrite MMD as:

$$MMD[\mathcal{F}, X, Y] := \|\mu_p - \mu_q\|_{\mathcal{H}} \quad (5.17)$$

Corollary 2. *Under the assumptions of theorem 1 the following is an unbiased estimator of $MMD^2[\mathcal{F}, p, q]$:*

$$MMD^2[\mathcal{F}, p, q] = \frac{1}{m(m-1)} \sum_{i \neq j}^{m} k(x_i, x_j) + \frac{1}{n(n-1)} \sum_{i \neq j}^{n} k(y_i, y_j) - \frac{2}{nm} \sum_{i,j=1}^{m,n} k(x_i, y_j) \quad (5.18)$$

5.8 Metrics Used in This Study

Naeem et al. [55] argue that the following are the necessary conditions for any useful evaluation metrics for generative algorithms:

1. Ability to detect identical real and fake distributions,

2. Robustness to outlier samples,

3. Responsiveness to mode dropping,

4. The ease of hyperparameter selection in the evaluation algorithms.

They believe that, even the most recent version of the precision and recall metrics (Kynkään-niemi, et al. [46]) fail to meet the requirements. Naeem et al. [55] introduced **Density** and **Coverage** metrics.

In this study, we aim to generate realistic synthetic ECG signals to address class-imbalance and enrich datasets. To achieve this, we propose the following necessary conditions for a set of synthetic ECG signals:

1. **Quality:** The synthetic beats should exhibit quality comparable to real beats, measured by their average distance (DTW, Fréchet distance functions) from an approved template.

2. **Distribution:** The distribution of the synthetic beats should closely resemble that of real beats, measured using the Maximum Mean Discrepancy (MMD)

3. **Equivalency:** The synthetic beats should be functionally equivalent to real beats in training a classifier, as assessed by the *Authenticity Test*

5.8.1 Quality: Average distance from an Approved Template

The *quality* of the generated synthetic beats are evaluated by comparing their average distance from an approved template with the corresponding value from the real beats.

After segmentation and normalization, the MIT-BIH Arrhythmia Database [52, 53] is transformed into a vector space:

$$\mathscr{V} = \{v_i^k\} \quad i = 1, \ldots, N^k \quad k = 1, \ldots, K \tag{5.19}$$

$$v_i^k = [v_{i,1}^k, \ldots v_{i,256}^k] \tag{5.20}$$

where v_i^k are the individual beats each with 256 (in the first and second papers) or 64 (in the third paper) timesteps, N^k is the number of beats in the class k, with K be the total number of classes.

The *approved template* for each class is denoted as $t^k = [t_{i,1}^k, \ldots t_{i,256}^k]$. A cardiologist selects a representative template from the real dataset for each class, ensuring that it encompasses all the pathological morphological patterns, features, and artifacts associated with that particular class.

The average distance of the synthetic beats in class k from an approved template is defined as:

$$d_{ave}^s = \frac{1}{N^k} \sum_{i=1}^{N_k} DF(v_i^k, t^k) \tag{5.21}$$

The corresponding value for the real beats from same class in the original dataset is:

$$d_{ave}^r = \frac{1}{N^k} \sum_{i=1}^{N_k} DF(r_i^k, t^k) \tag{5.22}$$

Obviously, if d_{ave}^s and d_{ave}^r are close, then, on the average basis, the generated data are at the same distance from the template as the real beats are.

5.8.2 Distributions

The second necessary condition which the synthetically generated beats should be evaluated against is their *distribution* which should be close to that of real data, if they are to augment the class-imbalanced dataset and create a balanced one [12]. Otherwise, new modalities will be added to the dataset. In simple terms, it has to be assured that the synthetic data have the same *mean* and *variance* as those of real data.

Maximum Mean Discrepancy (MMD) (Eq. 5.18) is the metric that can provide a quantitative measure for this purpose [12].

5.8.3 Authenticity or Equivalency

Authenticity test is used to evaluate if the synthetic beat are functionally equivalent to the real beats. In this test, **ResNet34** model has been used as the classifier which simulates a simplified automatic heart condition diagnosis machine.

Classifier: ECGResNet34

Network depth is of crucial importance on the performance of the model and the leading researches [34, 42, 69, 70] on the challenging *ImageNet* dataset [64] all exploit *very deep* models with typical depths of sixteen [69] to thirty [42] layers. On the flip side of the significance of depth, is the problem of *vanishing/exploding gradients* [9, 25, 39], which impedes convergence significantly. In fact the main question is: Is *bettering networks* as easy as just *stacking more layers* on top of each other?

One approach to address this problem is *normalized initialization* [25, 34, 47, 68] and *intermediate normalization layers* [42] which enables the deep networks which have convergence issues otherwise, start to converge using stochastic gradient descent with back-propagation.

He *et al.* [35] proposed a *deep residual learning frame work*, ResNet34, in which, they incorporate the *residual* mapping by introducing a repeating *building block* formulated as $\mathcal{F}(x) + x$, which represents a feed-forward neural network with *shortcut connections*(Fig. 5.7). The shortcut connections are basically an identity mapping network and skip one or more layers. Their outputs (which is identical to their input) is simply added to the output of the stacked layers, just in case the gradient has been *forgotten* (gradient vanishing) or *exaggerated* (gradient explosion) in passing through the stacked layers. The identity shortcuts do not add any computational complexity or extra training parameters to the model.

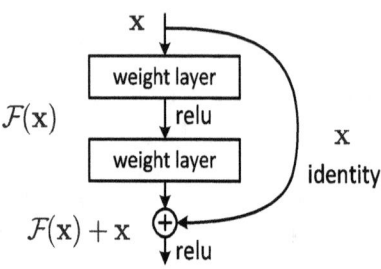

Figure 5.7: ResNet Building Block [35]

The formulation of the building block shown in Fig. 5.7 is:

$$y = \mathcal{F}(x, \{W_i\}) + x \qquad (5.23)$$

where x and y are the input and output of the block, respectively, and $\mathcal{F}(x, \{W_i\})$ represents the residual mapping to be learnt. For instance, for the block shown in Fig. 5.7 with two layers $\mathcal{F} = W_2 \sigma(W_1 x)$ in which σ denotes RelU. The dimension of x must be equal to that of $\mathcal{F}$, otherwise, a linear projection W_s can be used to match the dimensions:

$$y = \mathcal{F}(x, \{W_i\}) + W_s x \qquad (5.24)$$

This is not only attractive in practice but also important in comparing between *plain* and *residual* networks. We can fairly compare plain/residual networks that simultaneously have the same number of parameters, depth, width, and computational cost (except for the negligible element-wise addition).

ResNet34 is the state-of-the-art tool used in the classification of images. It has 34 layers along with the building blocks. Each block is comprised of two 3 × 3 convolutional layers with a residual stream. It is pretrained on the ImageNet dataset (more than 100, 000 images in 200 classes).

We used its *1D* implementation ([48]) to classify the heartbeats.

In Figure 5.8-Left, the VGG-19 model [69] (19.6 billion FLOPs) as a reference is shown. In the middle, a plain network with 34 parameter layers (3.6 billion FLOPs) is represented and in the right, a residual network with 34 parameter layers (3.6 billion FLOPs) is shown. The dotted shortcuts increase dimensions.

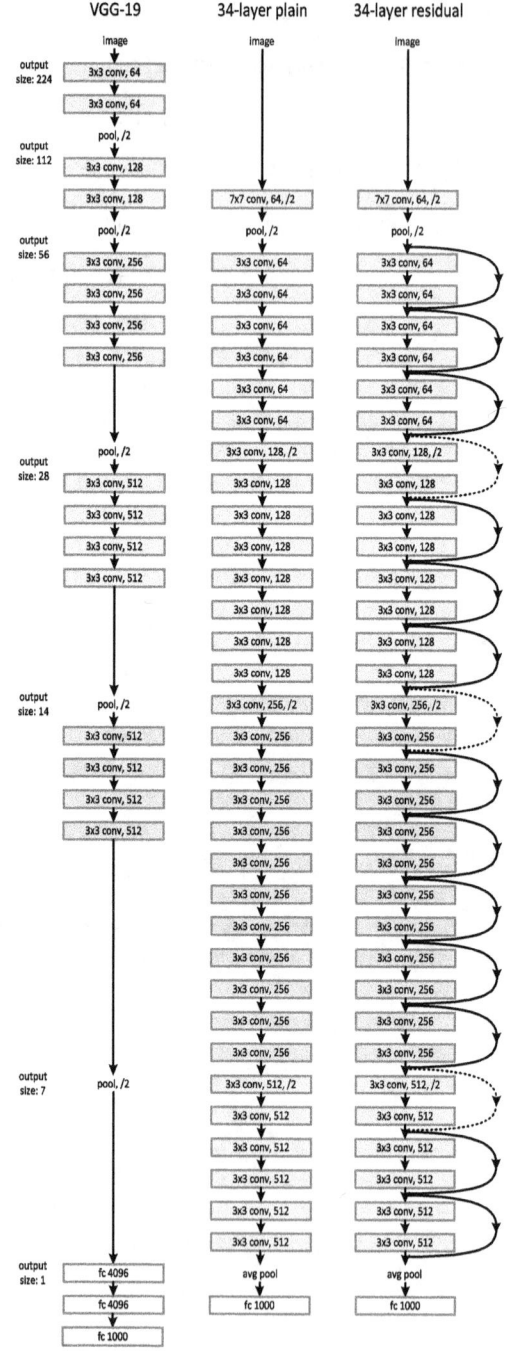

Figure 5.8: Example network architectures for ImageNet.

CHAPTER 6: *(PAPER 1)*
SYNTHETIC ECG SIGNAL GENERATION USING GENERATIVE NEURAL NETWORKS

6.1 Motivation

Cardiovascular diseases are one the major causes of death (for example, 31% of all deaths in 2016) [78]. Electrocardiogram (ECG) analysis is routine in any complete medical evaluation, mostly due to the fact that it is painless, noninvasive, and can easily reveal arrhythmia. The classification and diagnosis of arrhythmias is usually done by human experts of the domain, which is time consuming and prone to human error. Therefore, automatic ECG analysis and diagnosis is becoming of crucial importance more and more day by day. Classical supervised machine-learning shallow algorithms have been employed extensively for the classification of abnormalities in ECG ([22, 83, 84]). Deep learning unsupervised algorithms have also been successfully used as automatic diagnosis models and reached state-of-the-art results, reducing or eliminating the need for external feature engineering [4].

One of the challenges in the application of ML/DL algorithms on ECG is that their training datasets are usually highly *class-imbalanced* (e.g., see Figure 3.2), i.e., with regards to the number of samples per class, which causes the models perform poorly, especially on minor classes where there are not enough samples and the classifier cannot learn how to pick up the pattern [54].

Moreover, collected ECG data are sometimes noisy and accompanied with different types of artifacts, which may render some samples unusable or require pre-processing [59]. On the other hand, in spite of transfer learning, ML/DL algorithms generally still require huge and rich datasets for training. All these challenges suggest and justify the need for more synthetic ECG data and richer and larger artificially augmented and balanced datasets.

Another issue that justifies the need for synthetic ECG beat generation is *privacy*. Under various data protection and privacy laws, such as the General Data Protection Regulation (GDPR) in Europe or the Health Insurance Portability and Accountability Act (HIPAA) in the United States, health-related data, including ECG signals, is generally classified as sensitive personal information. As such, it is subject to strict regulations to ensure its proper handling, storage, and protection. [40].

To address all these issues, the generation of synthetic ECG signals has been the focus of many studies ([16, 26, 74, 79, 86, 88]).

6.2 Overview

The main objective of this paper [1] is to assess the capability of 5 models from the GAN family in generating synthetic Normal ECG heartbeats. This is an unconditional GAN model study, meaning that only one class data from the dataset has been used, both in training the generative model and in generating synthetic ECG beats.

Additionally, we collected and listed 5 different statistical methods to systematically evaluate the performance of the models in generating synthetic ECG beats. Since there is no consensus in the evaluation metrics for generative DL models, the models are compared on a case-by-case and application basis. These statistical methods, although not innovative, each present one aspect of averaging ans comparison. To measure the similarity (distances) between the beats, three similarity measures were incorporated: *Dynamic Time Warping* (DTW), *Fréchet*, and *Euclidean* distance functions.

6.3 Comparative Analysis to Previous Studies

This study is different from previous works ([16, 74, 88]) in that: *(i)* we employed more models from the GAN family in our comparison, *(ii)* we specifically incorporated WGAN, *(iii)* we used *lead-I* from the two available leads in the MIT-BIH Arrhythmia Dataset, ([16] used *lead-II*), and *(iv)* we present a systematic way to evaluate the performance of the models in generating synthetic data. *(v)* We devised a test to evaluate the *authenticity* or *realness* of the generated beats, which quantitatively measures how the generated beats can function as real beats do.

In addition, we introduce three new concepts: *threshold, acceptable beat, and productivity rate*. ***Thresholds*** are used to mathematically define ***acceptable beats*** as well as screen the generated

Table 6.1: Comparison with Major Related Works - I

Ref.	Year	Main Objective	GAN Variant	Arch. (Gen. Discr.)	Dataset
Delaney et al. [16]	2019	Generating Realistic Synthetic ECG Signal	Regular	LSTM-4CNN, BiLSTM-4CNN	MIT-BIH (Lead II)
Wang et al. [73]	2019	Dataset Augmentation/Balancing	ACGAN	14CNN-16CNN	MIT-BIH (Lead II)
Zhu et al. [88]	2019	Realistic Synthetic ECG	Regular	BiLSTM-(2CNN+FC)	MIT-BIH (one lead)
Zhang et al. [86]	2021	Synth ECG Generation	Regular	2D BiLSTM 5CNN-2D 4CNN FC	12 lead, PTB-XL, CCDD, CSE, Chapman
Wulan et al. [79]	2020	Realistic Synthetic ECG	DCGAN	2D 4TrCNN-2D 4CNN (SpectroGAN)	MIT-BIH (Lead I[1])
			Regular	2D 3FC-2D 3FC (WaveletGAN)	
This Study	2021	Realistic Synthetic ECG	Regular, WGAN	FC-FC, DC-DC, BiLSTM-DC, AE/VAE-FC, DC-DC (WGAN)	MIT-BIH (Lead I)

Table 6.2: Comparison with Major Related Works - II

Ref.	Multiclass Study/model	Mode Collapse Prevention	Metrics	Pre-Processing	No. of Epochs
Delaney et al. [16]	No/No (only Normal)	MBD [1] didn't work	MMD [2], DTW	Concatenation of beats	60
Wang et al. [73]	Yes/Yes	BN [3], DO [4]	ED, PCC [5], KL Div.	NM	150
Zhu et al. [88]	NM [6]	DO	PRD [7] RMS, FD [8]	NM	NM
Zhang et al. [86]	Yes/No	NM	MMD (IQR [9] SK [10] KU [11])	FWS [12]	up to 1000
Wulan et al. [79]	Yes/Yes	IN [13]	SVM [14], GTrTs [15]	4 second segmentation	NM
This Study	No/No	BN, Visual Inspection	Original Methods	Pan-Tompkins	30

beats for those that are low quality. We suggest a way to compute the threshold as well and we believe the ***productivity rate*** is a reasonable key indicator in the evaluation of performances. Also, the devised *authenticity* test, which is a binary classification model trained on synthetic datasets, shows that the augmentation of imbalanced datasets with synthetically generated ECG beats can improve the performance of classification comparably with the all real balanced dataset.

Tables 6.1, 6.2 and 6.3 compares this study with most prominent previous related researches.

Table 6.3: Comparison with Major Related Works - III

Ref.	Batch Size	Optimization	Learning Rate	Hyper-Parameter Fine-Tuning
Delaney et al. [16]	NM	Adam	NM	NM
Wang et al. [73]	NM	Adam	0.0001 (G) 0.0002 (D)	NM
Zhu et al. [88]	NM	NM	NM	NM
Zhang et al. [86]	32	NM	NM	NM
[79]	NM	RMSProp	0.0001 (SectroGAN) 0.00015 (Wavelet-GAN)	NM
This Study	9	Adam	0.0002	Recommended Suggestions

6.4 Dataset and Segmentation

The MIT-BIH Arrhythmia Database [27, 53] dataset is one of the most common benchmarks for ECG signal analysis and is used in this study as well. This dataset includes 48 30-minute two-channel ambulatory ECG records from 47 subjects studied by the BIH Arrhythmia Laboratory between 1975 and 1979. The recordings were digitized at 360 samples per second per channel with 11-bit resolution over a 10 mV range. This dataset is fully annotated with both beat-level and rhythm-level diagnoses. When segmented, the dataset is comprised of 109; 338 individual beats, of which 90; 502 beats are in the Normal class. See Chapter 3 for more details.

We borrowed the segmented dataset from Mousavi et al. [54] in this particular study. They used Pan-Tompkins segmentation method [58]. Their segmented beats are of the uniform length of 280, which were resampled to 256 in this study using the *scipy.signal.resample()* function:

$$\mathcal{V} = \{v_i^k\} \quad i = 1, \ldots, N_V^k \quad k = 1, \ldots, K \tag{6.1}$$

$$v_i^k = [v_{i,1}^k, \ldots v_{i,256}^k] \tag{6.2}$$

GAN Models Used

Mod.	Generator	Discriminator
01	Fully Connected (FC)	Fully Connected (FC)
02	Deep Convolutional (DC)	Deep Convolutional (DC)
03	BiLSTM	Deep Convolutional (DC)
04	Variational Autoencoder (VAE)	Deep Convolutional (DC)
05	Wasserstein	Deep Convolutional, Critic

Figure 6.1: GAN Models Used

6.5.1 Classic GAN (01)

The Generator is comprised of a block comprised of an FC followed by a Leaky ReLU layer, after which three sets of blocks each comprised of an FC, a BN and a leaky RelU layer and finally a block comprised of an FC followed by a hyperbolic tangent layer.

The Discriminator is comprised of 3 blocks of FC each followed by a Leaky ReLU except for the last block in which a sigmoid is used instead as the activation function.

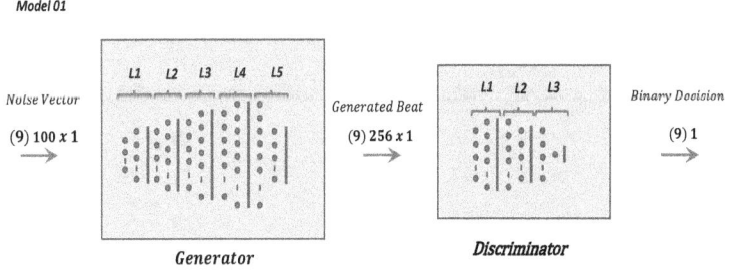

Figure 6.2: Model 01

Table 6.4: Classic GAN (01)

Layer	Generator	Discriminator
1	FC(100x128), L-ReLU(0.2)	FC(256x512), L-ReLU(0.2)
2	FC(128x256), BN, L-ReLU(0.2)	FC(512, 256), L-ReLU(0.2)
3	FC(256x512), BN, L-ReLU(0.2)	FC(256,1), sigmoid
4	FC(512, 1024), BN, L-ReLU(0.2)	-
5	FC(1024, 256), tanh	-

6.5.2 DC-DC GAN (02)

The Generator is comprised of five blocks, each includes a 1D Transposed Convolution, a BN and a Leaky ReLU layer. After these five blocks comes an FC followed by a hyperbolic tangent layer.

The discriminator is comprised of one 1D convolution followed by a Leaky ReLU, 3 blocks of 1D convolution followed by BN followed by a Leaky ReLU and finally comes one block of 1D convolution followed by an FC followed by a Leaky ReLU. The details are shown in Table 6.5 and in Figure 6.3 and 6.4.

Table 6.5: DC-DC GAN (02)

Layer	Generator	Discriminator
1	ConvTr1d(100x512), BN, L-ReLU(0.2)	Conv1d(1, 64), L-ReLU(0.2)
2	ConvTr1d(512, 256), BN, L-ReLU(0.2)	Conv1d(64, 128), BN, L-ReLU(0.2)
3	ConvTr1d(256, 128), BN, L-ReLU(0.2)	Conv1d(128, 256), BN, L-ReLU(0.2)
4	ConvTr1d(128, 64), BN, L-ReLU(0.2)	Conv1d(256, 512), BN, L-ReLU(0.2)
5	ConvTr1d(64, 1), BN, L-ReLU(0.2)	Conv1d(512, 1), FC(13, 1), sigmoid
6	FC (64, 256), tanh	-

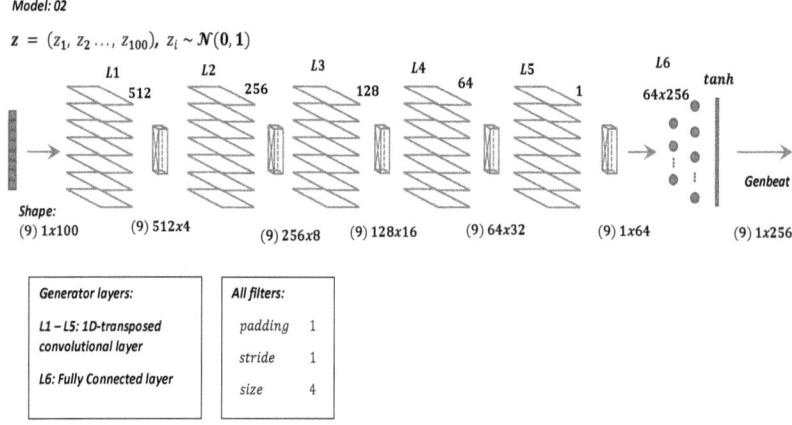

Figure 6.3: Model 02 (Generator)

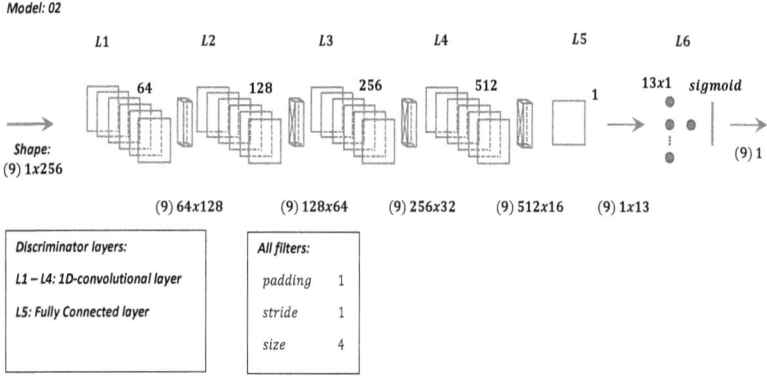

Figure 6.4: Model 02 (Discriminator)

6.5.3 BiLSTM-DC GAN (03)

In BiLSTM-DC GAN, a multi-layer *Bidirectional Long-Short Term Memory* block is used in the generator. The Discriminator block is almost the same as in DC-DC GAN. The details are shown in Table 6.6 and in Figure 6.5.

Table 6.6: BiLSTM-DC GAN (03)

Layer	Generator	Discriminator
1	BiLSTM(100, 1000), 2 layers	Conv1d(1, 64), L-ReLU(0.2)
2	FC(1000*2, 256), tanh	Conv1d(64, 128), BN, L-ReLU(0.2)
3	-	Conv1d(128, 256), BN, L-ReLU(0.2)
4	-	Conv1d(256, 512), BN, L-ReLU(0.2)
5	-	Conv1d(512, 1), FC(13, 1), sigmoid

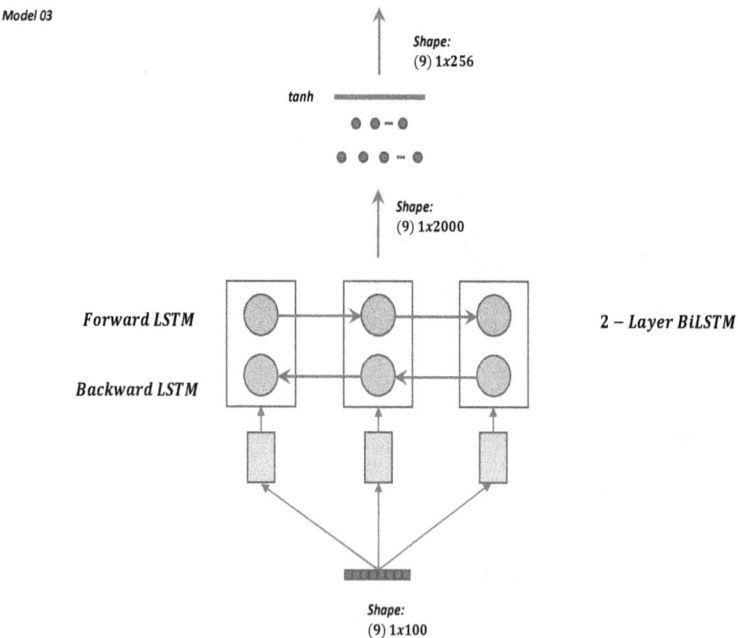

Figure 6.5: Model 03

6.5.4 AE/VAE-DC GAN (04)

In AE/VAE GANs, first a *real* sample from the dataset is fed to the encoder, where after passing through an FC layer followed by a Leaky-ReLU layer, it passes through a set of FC, a BN and

Leaky-ReLU layers. The output from these layers is a latent vector (bottleneck), x, which is the reduced dimension and condensed form of the *real* input. In AE version, this vector is the final output from the encoder. In fact, in AE, the input is mapped into the latent vector x. However, in VAE, this vector is transformed through reparameterization technique into a *multivariate probability distribution* which adds stochasticity into the process. In VAE, instead of directly feeding the reduced dimension vector x to the encoder, a sample is taken from the distribution and fed to the encoder. The reparameterization trick, makes the decoder much less sensitive to the small variations in the latent vector.

In reparameterization two other vectors, namely mean (μ) and variance (σ) are produced using the vector x as input which form a probability distributions. A random sample z is then drawn from this distribution as the output of the encoder. In this experiment only a Variational Autoencoder (VAE) GAN is used.

The original input is constructed back in the decoder. The random vector z (bottleneck) is used in the discriminator to discriminate between real and fake data.

Generator Loss - The bottleneck vector, Z, is fed to the discriminator and its output is fed to a Binary Cross Entropy (BCE) loss function where it is compared with an all-one vector, as the generator tries to fool the discriminator. Then the output from the decoder, i.e. the generated beat, is compared in an L1-loss function with the corresponding input which has been mapped into Z. The former and the latter are weighted by 0.001 and 0.999 respectively and produce the generator loss.

Discriminator Loss - A freshly generated multivariate random vector drawn from the standard normal distribution, Z_N, is fed to the discriminator and the output is compared with an all-one vector in a BCE loss function. Then, The latent vector output from the encoder, Z, is fed to the discriminator where it is compared with an all-zero vector in a BCE loss as the discriminator is to label the generated beat as fake. The arrhythmic average of these two will be used as the discriminator loss.

The details of the architecture are shown in the Table 6.7 and in Figure 6.6 and 6.7.

Table 6.7: AE/VAE-DC GAN (04)

Layer	Encoder	Decoder	Discriminator
1	FC(256, 512), L-ReLU(0.2)	FC(10, 512), L-ReLU(0.2)	FC(10, 512), L-ReLU(0.2)
2	FC(512, 512), BN, BN, LReLU	FC(512, 512), BN, L-ReLU(0.2)	FC(512, 256), L-ReLU(0.2)
3 *(mu)*	FC(512, 10)	FC(512, 256), tanh()	FC(256, 1), sigmoid
4 *(logvar)*	FC(512, 10))	-	-
5 *(Output layer)*	Reparameterization (mu, logvar)	-	-

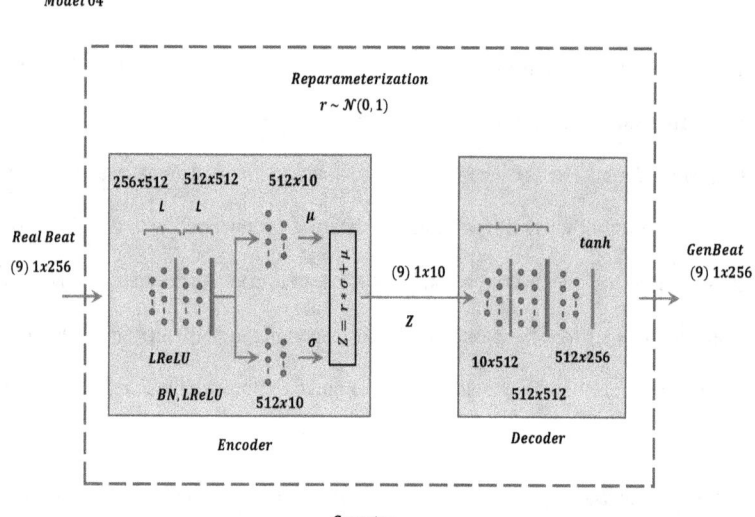

Figure 6.6: Model 04 (Generator)

model: 04

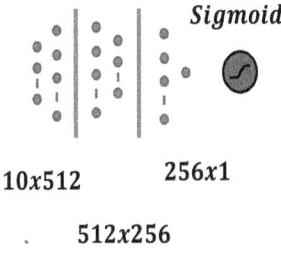

Figure 6.7: Model 04 (Discriminator)

6.5.5 WGAN (05)

The Generator has 6 blocks, each comprised of one 1D Transposed Convolution, a BN and a ReLU and finally a block of FC followed by a hyperbolic tangent activation.

In the discriminator, there are one block of 1D convolution plus a Leaky ReLU, 5 blocks of 1D convolution, BN and Leaky-ReLU and one 1D convolution as the last layer with no activation.

The Wasserstein distance (or *Earth-Movers*) function is incorporated. The details of the WGAN architecture is shown in Table 6.8 and in Figure 6.8 and 6.9.

Table 6.8: WGAN (05)

Layer	Generator	Discriminator
1	ConvTr1d(100x2048), BN, ReLU	Conv1d(1, 64), L-ReLU(0.2)
2	ConvTr1d(2048, 1024), BN, ReLU	Conv1d(64, 128), BN, L-ReLU(0.2)
3	ConvTr1d(1024, 512), BN, ReLU	Conv1d(128, 256), BN, L-ReLU(0.2)
4	ConvTr1d(512, 256), BN, ReLU	Conv1d(256, 512), BN, L-ReLU(0.2)
5	ConvTr1d(256, 128), BN, ReLU	Conv1d(512, 1024), BN, L-ReLU(0.2)
6	ConvTr1d(128, 64), BN, ReLU	Conv1d(1024, 2048), BN, L-ReLU(0.2)
7	Conv1d (64, 1), tanh	Conv1d(2048, 1)

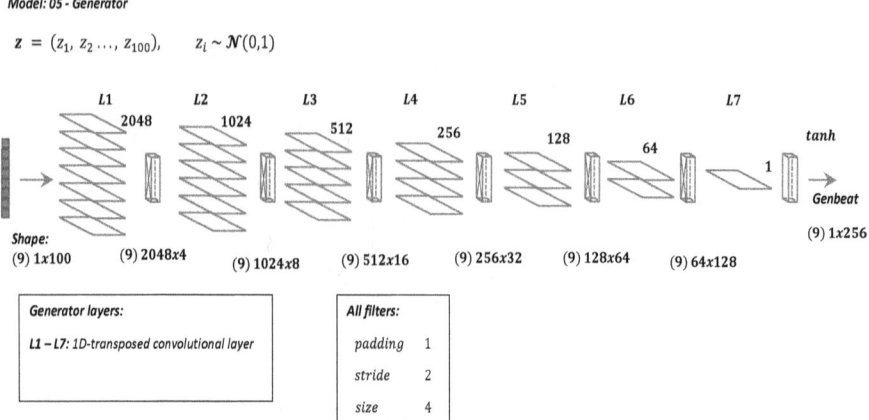

Figure 6.8: Model 05 (Generator)

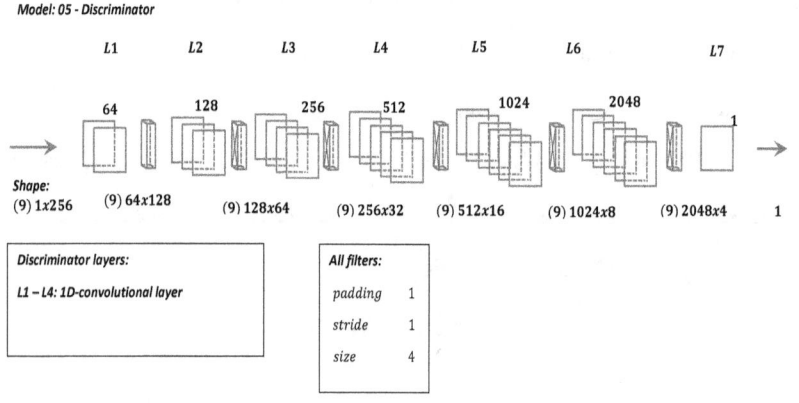

Figure 6.9: Model 05 (Discriminator)

6.5.6 Hyperparameter Settings

In all the models, the number of epochs is 30 with a batch size of 9. The optimizer used is ADAM with β_1 and β_2 equal to 0.5 and 0.999, respectively. The latent variable of a dimension of 100 is used at the generator input. Binary cross-entropy is used as the loss function. *Gaussian Normal Distribution* with a mean (μ) of 0 and a standard deviation (σ) of 0.02 is used for parameter initialization. In model 04 which is a hybrid model of VAE and GAN, the loss generator function is a weighted sum of the adversarial loss and the L_1 loss between the decoded beats and real beats.

6.6 Similarity Measures (Distance Functions)

Currently, there is a lack of consensus on the best evaluation metric for the performance of the generative models [15] and researchers mostly resort to the subjective expert-eye evaluation. In general, a distant function DF has a scalar output that quantifies the proximity (or distance) between its two input beats:

$$DF(\boldsymbol{x}, \boldsymbol{y}) : \mathscr{R}^{256} \times \mathscr{R}^{256} \to \mathscr{R} \tag{6.3}$$

6.6.1 Dynamic Time Warping (DTW)

DTW belongs to a family of measures known as *elastic dissimilarity measures* and it works by optimally aligning (warping) the time scale in a way that the accumulated cost of this alignment is minimal [10]. It constructs a cost matrix D based on the two time-series being compared, x and y. The elements of matrix D are defined, by a recurrent formula:

$$D_{i,j} = f(x_i, y_j) + \min\{D_{i-1,j}, D_{i,j-1}, D_{i-1,j-1}\} \tag{6.4}$$

for $i = 1, \ldots, M$ and $j = 1, \ldots, N$ where M and N are the lengths of the two time series $\boldsymbol{x}$ and $\boldsymbol{y}$. The local cost function $f(.,.)$ also called *sample dissimilarity function*, is usually the Euclidean distance. The final DTW value (distance or similarity) of the the time series $\boldsymbol{x}$ and $\boldsymbol{y}$ typically corresponds to the total accumulated cost, i.e., [10]:

$$d_{DTW}(\boldsymbol{x}, \boldsymbol{y}) = D_{M,N} \tag{6.5}$$

6.6.2 Fréchet Distance Function

If $P = (u_1, u_2, \ldots, u_p)$ and $Q = (v_1, v_2, \ldots, v_q)$ are two time series, a *coupling* L between P and Q is defined as the set of the links:

$$(u_{a_1}, v_{b_1}), (u_{a_2}, v_{b_2}), \ldots (u_{a_m}, v_{b_m}) \tag{6.6}$$

with $a_1 = 1$, $b_1 = 1$, $a_m = p$ and $b_m = q$, and for all $i = 1, \ldots, q$, $a_{i+1} = a_i$ or $a_{i+1} = a_i + 1$ and $b_{i+1} = b_i$ or $b_{i+1} = b_i + 1$. The length $\|L\|$ of the coupling L is defined as the longest (maximum Euclidean distance) in the link L:

$$\|L\| = \max_{i=1,\ldots,m} d(u_{a_i}, v_{b_i}) \tag{6.7}$$

Then the Fréchet distance between P and Q is defined as [7]:

$$d_{Fré} = \min\{\|L\| \mid L \text{ is a coupling between } P \text{ and } Q\} \tag{6.8}$$

6.6.3 Euclidean Distance Function

The Euclidean distance between two time series $P = (u_1, u_2, \ldots, u_n)$ and $Q = (v_1, v_2, \ldots, v_n)$ is defined as:

$$d_{Euc}(P, Q) = \sqrt{(u_1 - v_1)^2 + \cdots + (u_n - v_n)^2} \tag{6.9}$$

Fréchet distance function fulfills all the properties required by metric spaces (e.g., commutative, triangle property, ...) and can be used as a *metric*. However, DTW and Euclidean measures do not satisfy the triangle property and are not considered as metrics as required by metric spaces.

6.7 Templates

For each class, there is one template which is the quintessential time-series of that class and distinctly represents all the morphological features and patterns of the class. Distance functions take the template as well as a generated beat as inputs and generate a scalar number, which signifies the proximity of the two time-series. The following two approaches are available for developing/selecting templates.

6.7.1 Statistically Averaged Beat Template

Since all beats have an equal number of time steps (256), it is sensible that the template is defined as some sort of "mean of the class" such that the value at each time step is computed as the *mean* across all the beats of the class at that time step:

$$t = [\bar{v}_1, \ldots, \bar{v}_{256}] \tag{6.10}$$

$$\bar{v}_j = \frac{1}{N} \sum_{i=1}^{N_V} v_{i,j} \qquad j = 1, \ldots, 256 \tag{6.11}$$

N_V is the total number of samples (beats) in the set and t is the template. One sample of the template generated in this way is shown in Figure 6.10.

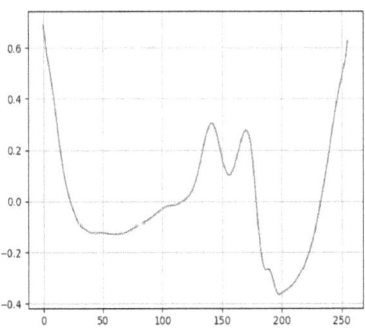

Figure 6.10: Statistically Averaged Template

6.7.2 Expert-Eye Selected Template

In this approach, the original dataset is visually inspected by a domain expert to find the "most fit sample" that meets all the morphological characteristics of that class. In this experiment, the expert-eye approach is employed to select the template, which is shown in Figure 6.11.

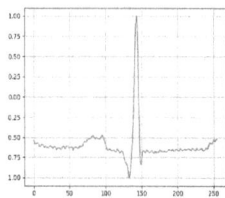

Figure 6.11: Selected Template

6.8 and Evaluating the Generated Beats

Evaluating the quality of the generated beats and the comparison between the performances of the models can be accomplished through one of the following four methods.

6.8.1 Method 1

the set of generated beats should be *close* to the set of the original dataset. To evaluate the proximity, the *whole set* of generated beats should be cross-compared to the *whole original dataset*, element by element. The outcome of this analysis, the mean, is a deterministic single number (with no randomosity) representing the average distance between the two sets. If $\mathcal{V}$ is the dataset space and $\mathcal{G}$ is the generated beats space, i.e.,:

$$\mathcal{G} = \{g_i\} \qquad i = 1, ..., N_G \qquad (6.12)$$

$$g_i = [g_{i,1}, ..., g_{i,256}] \qquad (6.13)$$

Then, the average distance between the two sets, d_{ave}^{DF}, is:

$$s_1^{DF} = d_{ave}^{DF} = \frac{1}{N_V N_G} \sum_{i=1}^{N_V} \sum_{j=1}^{N_G} DF(v_i, g_j) \qquad (6.14)$$

where DF can be DTW, $Fré$ or Euc distance function.

However, this analysis requires tremendous computational power. To approximate, one can instead apply Eq. 6.14 on two randomly selected *portions* from the two sets with sizes N_V^* and N_G^*. Of course, the method of sampling plays a significant role on the outcome and makes this process *stochastic*. The size of the portions depends on the available computational power (the more, the more accurate). In this experiment, we used $N_G^* = 300$ generated beats from each model (10 beats from each of the 30 epochs) and cross-compared them against $N_V^* = 300$ randomly selected beats from the original dataset. (Table 6.9).

Table 6.9: Method 1 (Portions of the Two Sets Compared with each other)

Model	Model	s_1^{DTW}	$s_1^{Fré}$	s_1^{Euc}
01	Classic GAN	*3.953*	*0.589*	8.325
02	DC-DC GAN	5.313	0.862	9.390
03	BiLSTM-DC GAN	4.535	0.625	8.557
04	AE/VAE-DC GAN	4.357	0.622	*8.230*
05	WGAN	4.401	0.681	8.486

6.8.2 Method 2

In this approach, the template is randomly selected from the original dataset and all the generated beats are compared with it. The average distance of all generated beats from the template is the score for that model:

$$s_2^{DF} = \frac{1}{N_G} \sum_{i=1}^{N_G} DF(v_i, t) \qquad (6.15)$$

This method is also obviously *stochastic*, as the outcome depends on the initial choice of the template. However, there is a constraint on the selected template which must have all the morphological features required by the class. Therefore, the variation is very limited and the results are more reliable. To select the best model, the scores are compared with each other in Table 6.10.

Table 6.10: Method 2 (All Beats Compared with One Template, Averages)

Model	Model	s_2^{DTW}	$s_2^{Fré}$	s_2^{Euc}
01	Classic GAN	**4.13**	0.595	8.44
02	DC-DC GAN	5.66	0.863	9.75
03	BiLSTM-DC GAN	4.33	*0.594*	*8.29*
04	AE/VAE-DC GAN	4.52	0.627	8.34
05	WGAN	4.59	0.693	8.71

6.8.3 Method 3

In this method, a template is randomly selected from the original dataset as in Method 2. Then, all the beats generated by each model are measured against the template and the beat which has produced the *minimum distance* value is reported as the "best beat" for that model. The score of the model is the distance of the best beat of that model with the template. This method measures the ultimate power of each model in getting as close to the template as possible (Table 6.11):

$$v_{best}^{DF} = \underset{v_i \in \mathcal{V}}{\arg\min} \, DF(v_i, t) \qquad (6.16)$$

$$s_3^{DF} = DF(v_{best}^{DF}, t) \qquad (6.17)$$

Table 6.11: Method 3 (Best Generated beat - Minimum Distance Functions)

Model Number	Model	s_3^{DTW}	$s_3^{Fré}$	s_3^{Euc}
01	Classic GAN	0.510	**0.0844**	0.890
02	DC-DC GAN	0.505	0.120	1.38
03	BiLSTM-DC GAN	0.425	0.0966	3.42
04	AE/VAE-DC GAN	0.505	0.108	1.02
05	WGAN	**0.311**	0.0981	**0.610**

6.8.4 Method 4

In this method a *threshold* is defined for each similarity measure (η^{DF}). Any generated beat (g_i) with a distance function value less than the threshold is considered as an *acceptable beat*, with respect to that distance function, i.e.,:

$$\mathscr{G}^{acc,DF} = \{g_i : DF(g_i, t) \leq \eta^{DF} \quad i = 1, ..., N_G\} \quad (6.18)$$

$$N_G^{acc,DF} = n(\mathscr{G}^{acc,DF}) \quad (6.19)$$

where $n(.)$ is number of the element in the set. Then the *Productivity Rate* (i.e. the percentage of the acceptable beats among all the generated beats) is calculated as the discriminating factor between the models:

$$s_4^{DF} = Prod^{DF} = \frac{n(\mathscr{G}^{acc,DF})}{n(\mathscr{G})} = \frac{N_G^{acc,DF}}{N_G} \quad (6.20)$$

The model which produces the highest productivity rate is the selected as the best in performance (Table 6.12).

The choice of the value of the threshold is rather arbitrary, experience-based and must be validated by an expert of the domain. It can be set at a factor of the minimum distance:

$$\eta^{DF} = a\, s_3^{DF} \qquad a \in \mathcal{R} \qquad (6.21)$$

In this experiment, for each distance function separately, it is basically computed as the arithmetic mean between the *minimum* and the *average* of the values of that particular distance function among all the generated beats:

$$\eta^{DF} = \frac{s_3^{DF} + s_2^{DF}}{2} \qquad (6.22)$$

Table 6.12: Method 4 (Productivity - Percent of Acceptable Beats, above threshold)

Model	Model	s_4^{DTW}	$s_4^{Fré}$	s_4^{Euc}
01	Classic GAN	**72.3**	**60.0**	10.5
02	DC-DC GAN	26.8	18.6	*11.2*
03	BiLSTM-DC GAN	54.2	47.0	0.437
04	AE/VAE-DC GAN	49.7	37.7	9.80
05	WGAN	49.0	38.05	8.50

6.8.5 Method 5

In this method, an expert with the domain-specific knowledge looks at the entire set of generated beats and gives their subjective judgment on the performance of the model. This is accomplished by inspecting the existence of the morphological features of the beat class in the set of generated beats.

6.8.6 Authenticity or Equivalency Test

We use the *Authenticity* or *Equivalency* test as a metric to show if augmentation of imbalanced dataset with synthetic ECG signals is effective or not.

- A subset of the MIT-BIH Arrhythmia dataset is selected which contained only two classes: N (Normal Sinus Beats) and L (Left Bundle Branch Block)

- A state-of-the-art classifier (***ECGResNet34***) [48] is trained on a balanced binary real dataset (L: 6455 and N: 6457). Its performance in classification is measured by recording the standard classification metrics: Precision, Recall, F1, Confusion Matrix. This is the *reference case* and all the *augmented* cases is compared with this case, as the synthetic beats should function as real beats.

- Some of the samples from class N is removed to create a *class-imbalanced* set. Then the classifier is trained on it. Obviously, the classifier cannot pick up the features and perform poorly, especially in the minor class, because there are not enough samples in class N.

- Now the *class-imbalanced* training set is augmented with synthetic beats so that the number of samples is exactly the same as the *reference case*. The synthetically generated beats are supposed to replace and function as real beats.

- 5 study cases is created as there are 5 set of synthetic data by the 5 models,

- The classifier is trained on the 5 augmented dataset and tested on the same unseen dataset as in the reference case,

The classifier is trained on each of these training sets and the classification metrics and confusion matrices are compared with each other in all the three cases. The test set (*unseen* data) is the same in all three cases (L: 1607 and N: 1609). The classifier used is ResNet34 [35] which is a 34-layer model and is the state-of-the-art in classification of images (2D). It incorporates residual building blocks following the residual stream logic: $F(x) + x$. Each building block is comprised of two

3×3 convolutional layers where the residual stream, x, goes directly from the input to the outlet of the block which prevents deterioration of training accuracy in deeper models [35]. We used its 1D implementation [48] to classify the heartbeats.

6.9 Platform and Code

A Dell Alienware with Intel i9-9900k at 3.6 GHz (8 cores, 16 threads) microprocessor, 64 GB RAM, and NVIDIA GeForce RTX 2080 Ti graphics card with 24 GB RAM, and also a personal Dell G7 laptop with an Intel i7-8750H at 2.2 GHz (6 cores, 12 threads) microprocessor, 20 GB of RAM, and NVIDIA GeForce 1060 MaxQ graphics card with 6 GB of RAM have been used in this study.

The codes were written in Python 3.8, and PyTorch 1.7.1 was used as the main deep learning network library. The codes are available on the GitHub page of the paper (`https://github.com/mah533/Synthetic-ECG-Generation---GAN-Models-Comparison`).

6.10 Results and Discussion

6.10.1 Templates and Typical Normal Beat

A statistically-averaged beat template is shown in Figure 6.10. The downside to this method of *averaging* is, although, all the beats have the same number of time-steps, small horizontal shifts of morphological features in temporal axis are inevitable (for instance, as a result of segmentation process or heart rate variability). Consequently, in calculation of the mean values ($\bar{v}_j$), more often than not, not all the corresponding points are averaged together (because of the shift). Therefor, the generated template looks completely distorted and totally different from Normal beat. In other words, the morphological characteristic features of that class are not distinguishable visually anymore. However, it should not be forgotten that the *statistically-averaged* template is the best representative of information from all the samples in the class, on an average basis and from statistical aspect and it has been used in similar studies (e.g., [73]).

6.10.2 Generated Beats by Different Models

Some samples of the generated beats by different models are presented in Figures 6.12 to 6.16. Figures in columns (a), (b) and (c) are the generated beats by each model with minimum DTW, Fréchet and Euclidean distance functions, (i.e., v_{best}^{DTW}, $v_{best}^{Fré}$ and v_{best}^{Euc}) respectively. The calculated values of all three distance functions are shown on the plots as well for comparison. In column (d), a beat selected from the last batch of the last iteration in the last epoch, which in fact, represent *maximally trained models'* outputs. It can be seen that, after convergence, more training does not necessarily result in a better beat, neither in appearance nor in terms of quantitative proximity. Finally, a beat that is visually close enough to the template in terms of morphological features and selected by an expert is shown in column (e). Its corresponding distance function values are shown for comparison.

Classic GAN (01)

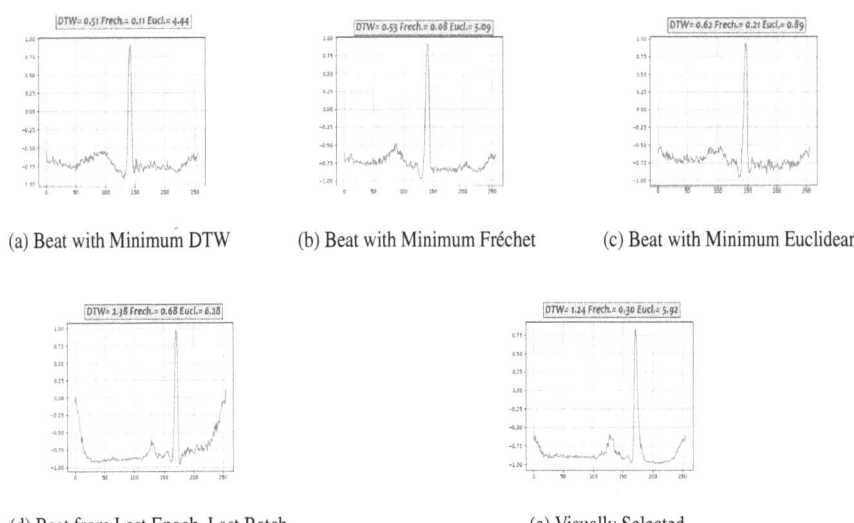

(a) Beat with Minimum DTW   (b) Beat with Minimum Fréchet   (c) Beat with Minimum Euclidean

(d) Beat from Last Epoch, Last Batch   (e) Visually Selected

Figure 6.12: Generated Beats, Classic GAN (01)

DC-DC GAN (02)

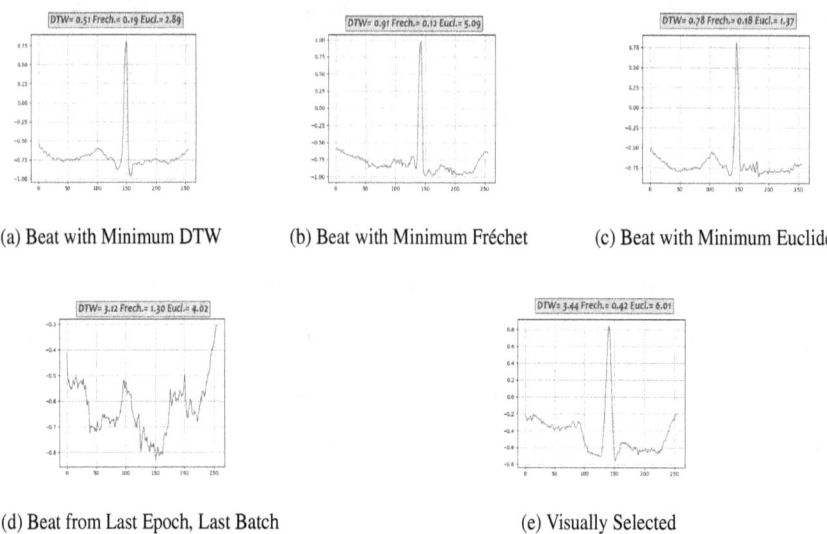

Figure 6.13: Generated Beats, DC-DC GAN (02)

BiLSTM-DC GAN (03)

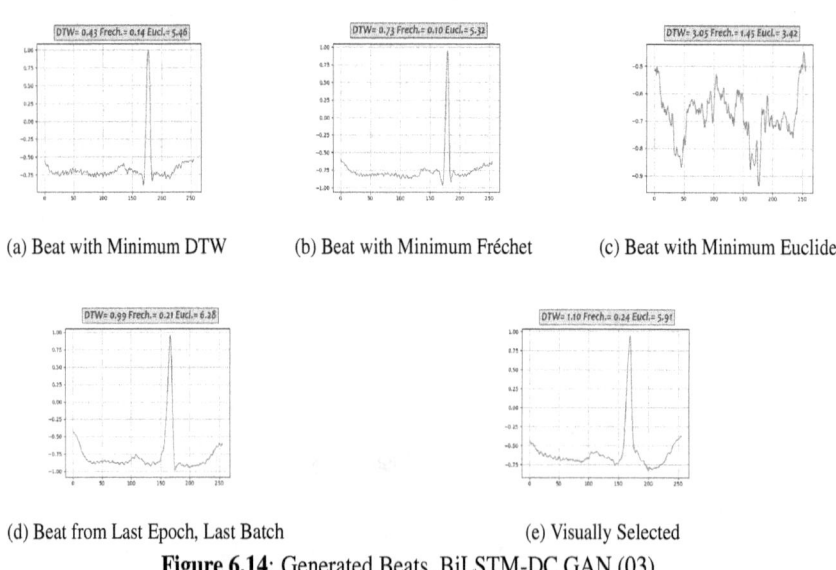

Figure 6.14: Generated Beats, BiLSTM-DC GAN (03)

DAE/VAE-DC GAN (04)

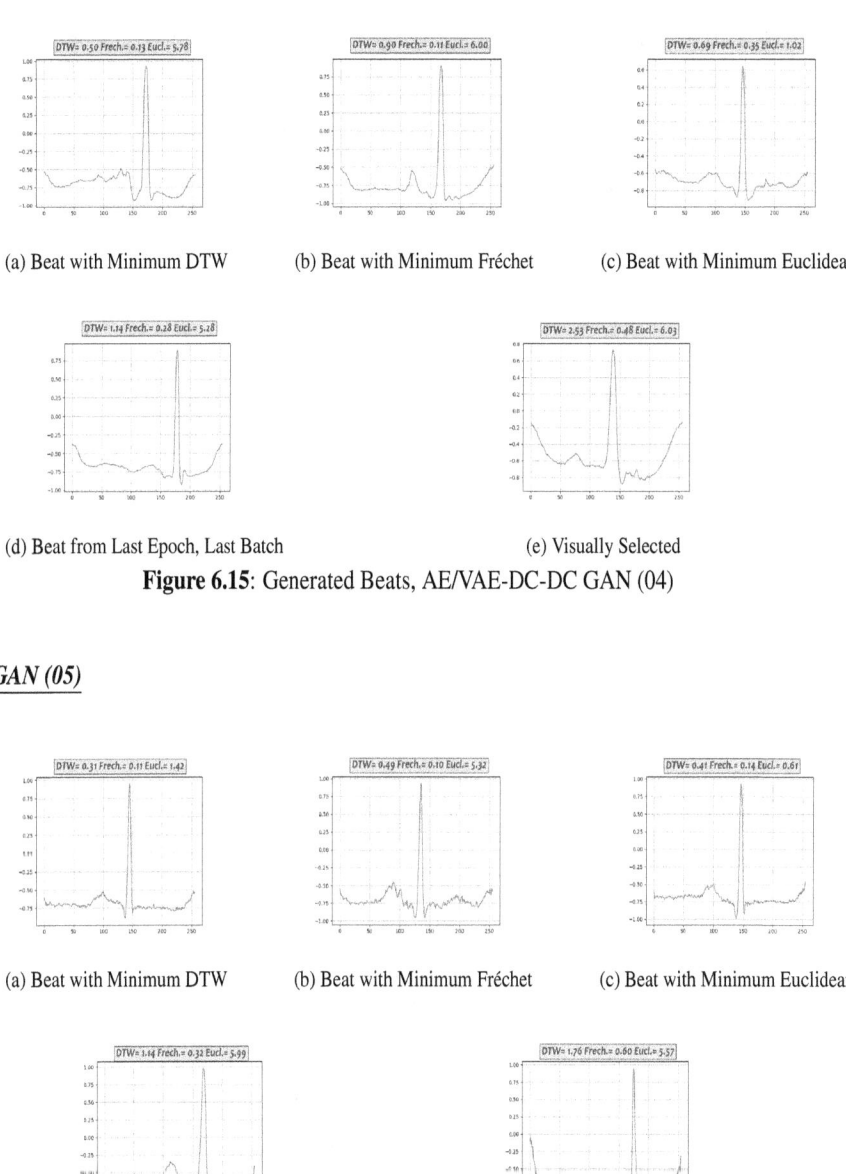

(a) Beat with Minimum DTW (b) Beat with Minimum Fréchet (c) Beat with Minimum Euclidean

(d) Beat from Last Epoch, Last Batch (e) Visually Selected

Figure 6.15: Generated Beats, AE/VAE-DC-DC GAN (04)

WGAN (05)

(a) Beat with Minimum DTW (b) Beat with Minimum Fréchet (c) Beat with Minimum Euclidean

(d) Beat from Last Epoch, Last Batch (e) Visually Selected

Figure 6.16: Generated Beats, WGAN (05)

6.10.3 Distance and Loss Functions

The trends of all three similarity measures as well as the generator and discriminator loss functions against the epoch number are plotted and shown in Fig 6.17. All graphs of the DC-DC GAN model (02) suffer from severe fluctuations, which is a result of a convergence issue. Fluctuation exists in other models as well, but they are not as severe.

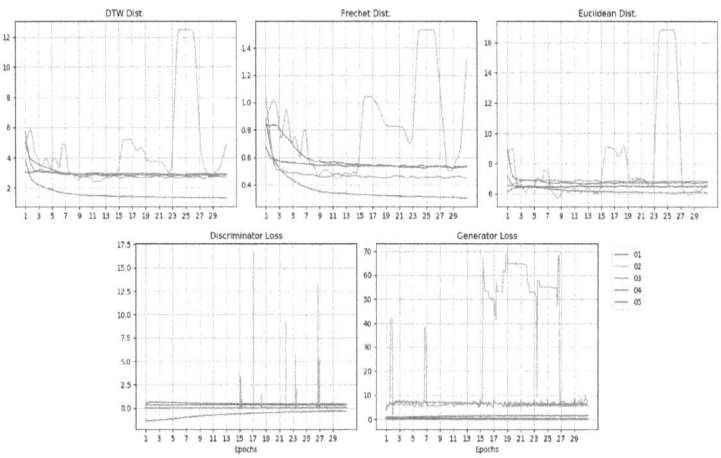

Figure 6.17: DTW Similarity Measure and Loss Functions vs Epoch Numbers

6.10.4 Performance Metrics

Table 6.9 summarizes the performance metrics s_1^{DTW}, $s_1^{Fré}$ and s_1^{Euc} of the five models. As shown, Classic GAN (in terms of DTW and Fréchet distance functions) and AE/VAE-DC GAN (in terms of the Euclidean distance function) seemingly generate synthetic sets of beats closest to the original dataset. However, it should be noted that this analysis is stochastic, as the outcome depends on the method of sampling, i.e. the way the portions are selected. Therefore, the resulting outcomes are basically just one realization of the corresponding random variables. Nevertheless, these numbers show that all the models are, give or take, in the same ballpark range.

Table 6.10 shows the result of the comparison using Method 2 (s_2^{DTW}, $s_2^{Fré}$ and s_2^{Euc}), i.e., the average distances from the template. Similar to Method 1, this process is also random because it depends on the choice of template. However, since the selected template is constrained to have all the morphological features of the class, the outcome numbers are much more reliable. The results show that with respect to the DTW distance function *Classic GAN*, with respect to Fréchet, both the *Classic GAN* and *BiLSTM-DC GAN* models equally, and with respect to Euclidean distance function *BiLSTM-DC GAN*, perform the best.

The result of the analysis using Method 3, (s_3^{DTW}, $s_3^{Fré}$ and s_3^{Euc}) (the distance of the best generated beat from the template), are shown in Table 6.11. The results show that in terms of DTW and Euclidean, *WGAN* perform the best, and in terms of Fréchet distance function, *Classic GAN* perform the best.

Assessment in terms of productivity rates (s_4^{DTW}, $4_2^{Fré}$ and s_4^{Euc}) method 4 , Table6.12), reveals that 72.3% and 60.0% of the generated beats by the *Classic GAN* (01) model are acceptable with respect to the DTW threshold ($\eta^D TW$) and Fréchet threshold, respectively. The Euclidean measure selects the *DC-DC GAN* with only 11% of success. This method, like Method 2, is essentially random, but since the selected template is constrained, its randomosity is very limited.

Visual inspection of the generated beats by a domain-expert knowledge (Method 5) suggests subjectively that *WGAN* and *BiLSTM-DC GAN* models produce more acceptable beats than the other models.

6.10.5 Authenticity Test and Efficacy of Augmentation

Comparing the results in Tables 6.14 and 6.15 shows that the augmentation of the imbalanced dataset with synthetically generated beats can improve the classification drastically, almost as in real balanced dataset Table 6.13. Same trend is noticeable from confusion matrices Tables 6.16 (a), (b) and (c).

Table 6.13: Classification Report, Real Data, Balanced

Class	Precision	Recall	F1-Score	Support
L	0.95	0.96	0.96	1609
N	0.96	0.95	0.95	1607
Accuracy	-	-	0.95	3216
Macro Avg	0.96	0.95	0.95	3216
Micro Avg	0.96	0.95	0.95	3216

Table 6.14: Classification Report, Real Data, Imbalanced

Class	Precision	Recall	F1-Score	Support
L	0.52	1.00	0.68	1608
N	1.00	0.08	0.15	1608
Accuracy	-	-	0.54	3216
Macro Avg	0.76	0.54	0.42	3216
Micro Avg	0.76	0.54	0.42	3216

Table 6.16: Confusion Matrices (all values are in %)

	N	L
N	85.7	14.3
L	5.4	94.6

(a) Real Data, Balanced

	N	L
N	37.1	62.9
L	28.2	71.8

(b) Real Data, Imbalanced

	N	L
N	73.6	26.4
L	21.0	79.0

(c) Augmented Data

6.11 Conclusion

Machine Learning automatic ECG diagnosis models classify ECG signals based on the morphological features within the beats. ECG datasets are usually highly class-imbalanced due to the fact that the *anomaly* cases are scarce compared to the abundant *Normal* cases. Additionally, ECG signals are considered private information and because of privacy concerns, not all the collected data from real patients are available as training sets. Therefore, it is necessary that realistic synthetic ECG signals can be generated and made publicly available.

Table 6.15: Classification Report, Augmented Data, Balanced

Class	Precision	Recall	F1-Score	Support
L	0.99	0.95	0.97	1607
N	0.95	0.99	0.97	1609
Accuracy	-	-	0.97	3216
Macro Avg	0.97	0.97	0.97	3216
Micro Avg	0.97	0.97	0.97	3216

In this study, we compared the efficiency of a few DL models in generating realistic synthetic ECG signals using 5 different methods from the Generative Adversarial Network (GAN) family. The 3 introduced concepts (threshold, accepted beat and productivity rate) are employed to systematically evaluate the models and can be used in end-to-end methods.

The results from using Method 1 in comparing models suggest that all the tested models compete very closely in generating synthetic ECG beats (Table 6.9). The fact that all the results are numerically in the same ballpark shows that, through this method (metrics s_1^{DTW}, $s_1^{Fré}$ and s_1^{Euc}), all models behave more or less equally well in generating acceptable beats.

What matters in generating synthetic beats for augmenting datasets is the *productivity rate* (s_1^{DTW}, $s_1^{Fré}$ and s_1^{Euc}), i.e., the efficiency of models in terms of time and computational power, which translates into the percentage of the acceptable beats. In fact, a good model is the one that generates more acceptable beats per unit of time and computational power. We believe the productivity rate (Method 4) is a very efficient way to assess the capability of models in end-to-end generation of the synthetic ECG signals.

Performance analysis using Method 4 shows that Classic GAN has the highest productivity rate in terms of the DTW distance function, whereas the percentages of the *BiLSTM-DC*, *AE/VAE-DC GAN*, and *WGAN* models are all slightly lower but in the same ballpark, and the productivity rate of the *DC-DC GAN* is the lowest. Fréchet distance function exhibits the same trend, although at slightly lower levels. Thus, using Method 4, *Classic GAN* has the highest percentage of acceptable beats and is the most efficient model with respect to the DTW and Fréchet similarity measures.

This might seem a bit counter-intuitive at first, but as FC architectures are very powerful mapping functions and can potentially simulate most complicated non-linearities and functions, they can map the latent space to real data space very well. The values of the Euclidean measure are so low altogether that it does not seem to be a suitable distance function for this purpose. For instance, Fig 6.14 (c) shows one generated beat with minimum Euclidean Distance whereas it contains none of the morphological features. The fact that both DTW and Fréchet distance functions show the same trend indicates that both are suitable measures for the comparison and the choice is just a matter of computational power. Visual inspection of the the generated beats (Method 5) shows that *BiLSTM-DC GAN* and *WGAN* generate acceptable beats more often than the others.

There is a lack of a systematic way for the performance assessment of models for generative models, contrary to classification tasks (in which the performance metrics are standardized), and the performance is measured in practice based on the quality and quantity of the generated data on a case-based basis. We believe Methods 1 to 4 can fill the gap and provide quantitative measures for assessments of GAN family models. Our simple experiment with the state-of-the-art classifier (ECGResNet34) showed empirically that the augmentation of imbalanced ECG dataset and balancing them with synthetic ECG signals can improve the classification performance drastically.

6.12 Future Works

A better similarity measure that can capture the similarity between time series more reliably and can eliminate the supervision of humans would help greatly.

Using different loss functions in the algorithms with various regularizations that can capture the difference between time series in a better way can result in a better convergence and alleviate fluctuations in error/loss functions.

CHAPTER 7: *(PAPER 2)*
ARRHYTHMIA CLASSIFICATION USING CGAN-AUGMENTED ECG SIGNALS

7.1 Overview and Contribution

Unconditional Generative Adversarial Network (Unconditional GAN) are trained only on one class of data. The trained generator is capable to generate synthetic data only in the same class. However, another approach to address class-imbalance in ECG datasets, is to utilize Conditional GAN (CGAN) models to generate realistic synthetic ECG signals. CGAN are trained on a number of classes at the same time, where, the input is conditioned on the *class*. Therefore, the trained generator is capable of generating synthetic data in many classes. The input latent variable to the generator is conditioned on class, so that the generator knows to which class the generated data should belong.

In this paper [2] we developed a 1D conditional GAN (AC-WGAN-GP) and applied it to generate ECG signals (single heartbeat time series) for the first time. We investigated the impact of data augmentation on the performance of classification of imbalanced datasets.

The MIT-BIH Arrhythmia dataset is used to train two models from the GAN family: *(a) unconditional GAN* (Wasserstein GAN with gradient penalty, WGAN-GP) and *(b)* the developed *conditional GAN* (Auxiliary Classifier Wasserstein GAN with gradient penalty, AC-WGAN-GP). In each case, the generated data are used in two scenarios: *(i) unscreened* or raw, i.e., without any further processing and *(ii) screened*, i.e., only a subset of generated beats is used: each generated beat was measured up against the corresponding template and discarded if its distance was above a certain threshold.

The models are compared by the *quality* of the generated beats which is measured by the average distance from an approved template. For reference, the quality of the *real* data from the MIT-BIH dataset is also measured.

Also, the synthetically generated data in each study case is evaluated for the *Authenticity*. In this test, which is utilized as a metric, the generated data are used to augment a class-imbalanced dataset and create a well balanced dataset. Then, the state-of-the-art classifier (*EcgResNet34*) was used to perform a classification task. The impact of augmentation is investigated by the standard classification metrics (micro-averaged Precision score, multi-class Precision-Recall curves and the *net improvement* in True Positives (confusion matrix' main diagonals)) and confusion matrix are used.

Generating synthetic ECG signals can provide a richer data set which is potentially expandable indefinitely, while the other options (new design of loss functions or new scheme of training) only soften the negative impact of imbalance in datasets. To the best of our knowledge, this is the first time that a *1D* AC-WGAN-GP model is developed and applied on the benchmark MIT-BIH dataset with the intention of enrichment of the dataset.

7.2 GAN Models

In general, generative models find the distribution of the original data either implicitly (e.g., in GAN models [29]) or explicitly (e.g., in V/AE models [18]).

As discussed in Section 4.4, GAN models are a comprised of two blocks of networks: the generator and the discriminator [29]. These two blocks compete in a two-player zero-sum game with a loss function of $V(G, D)$ (Eq. 4.13), where the generator tries to generate fake data so close to the original real data distribution that the discriminator cannot distinguish from the real data. The discriminator is a binary classifier that is trained on real and fake data to classify the inputs as real or fake.

The following types of GAN family are utilized in this study as described below:

7.2.1 WGAN-GP (Unconditional)

It can be shown that $V(G, D)$ in (4.13) reduces to Jensen-Shannon distance between the distributions of the real and fake data when the discriminator is at its optimum [6]. Jensen-Shannon distance function is not a smooth function and is not differentiable at zero, whereas the Wasserstein distance function, Eq. 4.14, has a smooth behavior and is differentiable everywhere. Moreover, it prevents the mode collapse which is a very common issue in regular GAN. All these lead to a better and more stable training.

The necessary condition of *k*-Lipschitz continuity is satisfied in WGAN by a technique called Parameter Clipping [6], i.e., keeping the magnitude of parameters of the model bounded, which can easily lead to vanishing/exploding gradient. In WGAN with gradient penalty (WGAN-GP) [31], the *k*-Lipschitz continuity constraint is satisfied by regularizing the loss function to keeping the norm of the gradient below 1.

7.2.2 AC-WGAN-GP (Conditional)

WGAN-GP is an unconditional model i.e., the probability distributions used in the loss function are not conditional. Thus, all the data (training and generated) are in one class. However, if the probabilities in the loss function in (4.13) are conditioned on the labels, the model becomes multiclass [31].

$$\min_{G} \max_{D} V(G, D) = E_{x \sim P_{data}(X)}[log D(X|y)] + E_{z \sim P_z(z)}[log(1 - D(G(z|y)))] \quad (7.1)$$

7.3 Dataset and Segmentation

The MIT-BIH Arrhythmia dataset (Chapter 3) is used in this study. However, the segmentation method is different from the previous study (see Section 3.9.2).

7.4 Designs of Models

Two models have been used to generate beats: *unconditional* GAN (WGAN-GP) and the developed *conditional* GAN (AC-WGAN-GP). WGAN is chosen because of its better behavior in training and mode collapsing prevention.

Unconditional GAN

The architectures of the generator and the critic are comprised of building blocks, which are repeated multiple times. In the generator they are comprised of: *(1)* 1D transpose convolution layer (ConvTranspose1d) with a kernel size of 4, a stride of 2 and padding of 1, *(2)* a 1D batch normalization (BatchNorm1d) and *(3)* a rectified linear unit (ReLU). In the critic they are comprised of: *(1)* a 1D convolutional layer with a kernel size of 4, a stride of 2 and padding of 1, *(2)* a 1D instance normalization layer (InstanceNorm1d), and *(3)* a Leaky ReLU (LeakyReLU). The details of the architectures are shown in Table 7.1. The numbers in the brackets are the dimensions of the output from the layer.

Table 7.1: Unconditional GAN Architecture

Layer	Generator	Critic
Input	$16 \times 100 \times 1$	$16 \times 1 \times 256$
1	Block	Vonv1d, LeakyReLU
2	Block	Block
3	Block	Block
4	Block	Block
5	ConvTranspose1d	Conv1d
6	FC (64, 256)	FC (64, 256)
7	tanh	-
Output	$16 \times 1 \times 256$	$16 \times 1 \times 1$

Conditional GAN

We combined 1D conditional GAN with WGAN-GP to develop *1D* version AC-WGAN-GP. Class labels are embedded to a dimension of (100×1) and concatenated with the latent variable with the same dimension before feeding to the generator. The concatenated input to the generator has a dimension of (200×1) (Figure 7.1). In the critic, the labels are embedded to a dimension of (1×256) and then concatenated to the heartbeat signal (fake or real) with the dimension of

(1×256) *as a channel* to produce an input of (2×256) befor being fed to the critic. The same building blocks in the generator and the critic of WGAN-GP are used correspondingly in this model too. The generator and critic parameters are initialized from a normal distribution with zero mean and a standard deviation of 0.02. The Adam optimizer was used with a learning rate of 0.0001. The details of the rest of the architectures are shown in Tables 7.2 and 7.3.

Table 7.2: Conditional GAN Architecture - Generator

Layer	Generator	
Input		16 (label)
1	$16 \times 100 \times 1$ (feature)	embedding (16×100)
2		reshape $(16 \times 100 \times 1)$
3	Concatenate $(16 \times 200 \times 1)$	
4	block $(16 \times 1024 \times 1)$	
5	block $(16 \times 512 \times 8)$	
6	block $(16 \times 256 \times 6)$	
7	block $(16 \times 128 \times 32)$	
8	ConvTranspose $(16 \times 1 \times 64)$	
9	FC (16×256)	
10	reshape $(16 \times 1 \times 256)$	
11	FC $(16 \times 1 \times 256)$	
12	$16 \times 1 \times 256$	

Table 7.3: Conditional GAN Architecture - Critic

Layer	Critic	
Input		16 (label)
1	$16 \times 1 \times 256$ (feature)	embedding (16×256)
2		reshape $(16 \times 1 \times 256)$
3	Concatenate $(16 \times 2 \times 256)$	
4	Conv1d, ReLU $(16 \times 64 \times 128)$	
5	block $(16 \times 128 \times 64)$	
6	block $(16 \times 256 \times 32)$	
7	block $(16 \times 512 \times 16)$	

2nd Paper:
Contribution

- Auxiliary Classifier WGAN with Gradient Penalty (AC-WGAN-GP)
  - "in 1D" is developed for the first time

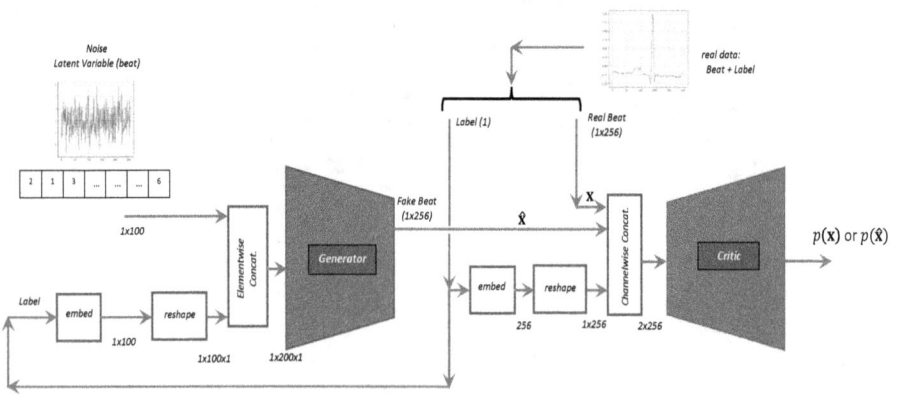

Figure 7.1: Architecture of Developed $1D$ Conditional WGAN-GP

7.5 Experimental Description

There are 15 classes altogether in the MIT-BIH dataset. We picked 7 classes, namely: **P** (Paced Beat), **A** (Atrial Premature Contraction), **L** (Left Bundle Branch Block Beat), **N** (Normal Beat), **R** (Right Bundle Branch Block Beat), **f** (Fusion of Paced and Normal Beat), **j** (Nodal/Junctional Escape Beat). The support sets of the selected classes are shown in Table 7.4. First, the data in each class are split randomly into the training and test sets by a split ratio of $0.9/0.1$. However, only 50% of samples in each class are actually used in training because we wanted the classifier to train on a highly imbalanced dataset and perform purposely poorly due to an insufficient number of samples in minor classes. The number of samples *actually* used in each set/class are also shown in Table 7.4. The classifier used is the state-of-the-art (*EcgResNet34*). It is trained on the imbalanced training set and the classification metrics were calculated. The metrics used are Precision/Recall/F1-score (per class, macro- and micro-averaged), total accuracy, confusion matrix, as well as Precision-Recall curve). This is our *reference case* and its metric results were compared with the corresponding values for all the four augmented study cases.

Table 7.4: Selected Classes From MIT-BIH Arrhythmia Dataset
Number of Samples

Cl.	Total	Samples Used (train set)	Samples Used (test set)
P	7028	3162	703
A	2546	1145	255
L	8075	3633	806
N	75052	33773	7500
R	7259	3266	726
f	982	441	99
j	229	103	23

7.5.1 Templates

For each class, a sample beat is selected visually by a domain expert as the template to represent the class. The template should have all the required patterns and morphological features which the domain expert determines.

Four Study Cases

The generated beats by the two models, i.e., *(a)* conditional and *(b)* unconditional GANs, are used once as *(i) raw* or *unscreened*, and once as *(ii) screened*. In the first scenario with *raw* signals, all the generated beats are used whereas in *screened* case, only the good quality beats are used, i.e., each generated beat is compared with the template of its class using the DTW distance function and discarded if its distance is greater than the threshold. Thus, four study cases were formed:

- *Case I*: Conditional GAN, raw generated beats

- *Case II*: Conditional GAN, screened generated beats

- *Case III*: Unconditional GAN, raw generated beats

- *Case IV*: Unconditional GAN, screened generated beats

Threshold and Distance Function

Dynamic Time Warping (DTW) is used as the distance function. It takes two heartbeat $1D$-vectors as inputs and generates a scalar which represent the distance between the two inputs. A threshold is used in screening as the cutoff. The threshold was around 1.5-2 for all classes except for class L which was 5. The reason for a higher threshold for class L is that the generated data in this class were so noisy and screening with such a tight margin threshold were extremely time-consuming.

7.5.2 Platform and Codes

For the machines and software used in this study (see Section 6.9).

The codes are available on the GitHub page of the paper (https://github.com/mah533/Augmentation-of-ECG-Training-Dataset-with-CGAN).

7.6 Results and Discussion

7.6.1 Samples of Generated Beats

A sample of the generated beats in each class is shown in Figure 7.2.

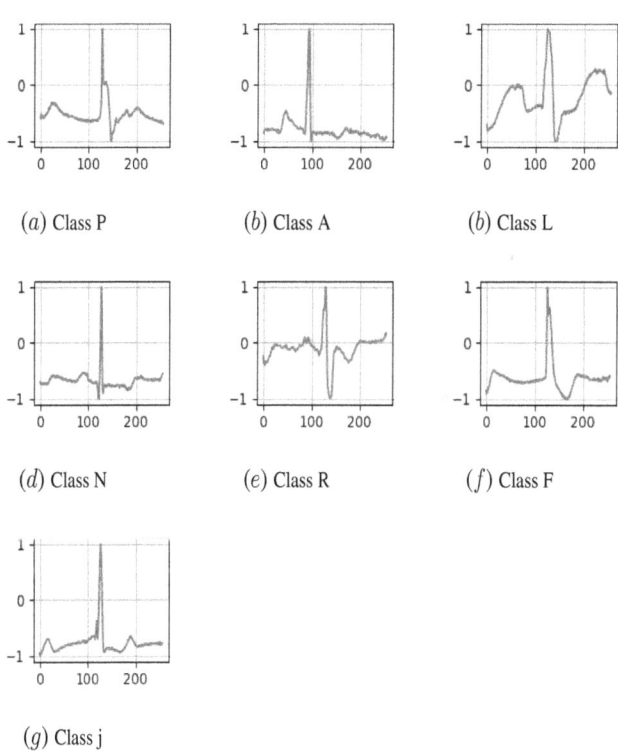

Figure 7.2: Samples of Generated Beats

7.6.2 Precision or Recall

In this study we are firstly interested in samples which can be classified correctly, i.e., maximizing number of true positives (TP). Secondly, we like to minimize number of false positives (FP), i.e., those samples which are mistakenly classified as correct. Thus, $\frac{FP}{TP}$ is to be minimized. Therefore, Precision score ($Pr = \frac{TP}{TP+FP} = \frac{1}{1+FP/TP}$) relates to the purpose of this study more than Recall score, as in the abundance of the generated data, it does not really matter if some of the *good* samples are overlooked (false negatives). However, Precision-Recall curve captures the trade-off between the two scores at different thresholds. Micro-averaged Precision scores favor **Case III** with the highest value of 0.97 (Table 7.12). Also, Precision-Recall curve selects **Case III** with highest area under the curve (Figure 7.3 (e)). Both scores are consistent with the Net Improvement score.

7.6.3 Quality of Generated Beats

Table 7.5 summarizes the quality of the generated beats in the *Cases I* through *IV* plus that of real data, quantified by the DTW distance function and expressed as the average distance from the template in each class. Unlike screened cases (*II* and *IV*), Raw cases (*I* and *III*) show DTW values relatively higher than those of the real data almost in all classes, which is quite reasonable because in the screened cases, all the *off* beats are discarded already. Evidently, the distribution of the set will change by the screening.

Table 7.5: Quality of Generated Beats & Real Data
Average DTW Distance from Template

Cl.	Case I (C.[1] Raw)	Case II (C. Screened)	Case III (U.[2] Raw)	Case IV (U. Screened)	Real Data
P	5.99	2.09	4.05	1.52	4.01
A	6.56	1.72	6.26	1.59	6.70
L	5.00	2.35	4.79	3.12	3.94
R	3.37	0.85	4.39	0.82	3.64
f	3.35	2.14	2.47	2.00	2.80
j	5.04	2.14	3.47	2.09	3.01

1: Conditional   2: Unconditional

7.6.4 Classification Results and Confusion Matrices

Reference Case

Figure 7.3 (a) shows the multiclass Precision-Recall curve for the reference case (imbalanced dataset). The classification report and the confusion matrix for this case are shown in Tables 7.6 and 7.7, respectively. Since the training set was highly imbalanced, the poor performance was predictable, especially in the minority classes ("f" and "j"). In class "j" only 1 sample out of 23 (4.35%) is classified correctly and in class "f", only 65.7% of samples are classified correctly, whereas in other classes where the number of samples was high enough, more samples are correctly classified which is reflected in the confusion matrix diagonals.

Augmented Training Sets (Cases I through IV)

The original imbalanced dataset is augmented with the generated synthetic beats in cases *I* through *IV* and each is balanced up to a total of 10,000 samples per class. Then the classifier *EcgResNet34* is trained on the four augmented datasets. The same unseen test set is used to evaluate the improvements achieved by augmentation in classification performances compared to the *Reference Case*. The classification metrics and the confusion matrix results for the four study cases are shown in Tables 7.8 to 7.15. Also the corresponding multiclass Precision-Recall curves are shown in Figures 7.3 (c) through (f).

The results show a uniform and significant improvement in all metrics in all cases. The same improvement is seen in the corresponding confusion matrix of all the four cases. The number of samples which are classified correctly, especially in minor classes, improved significantly.

Table 7.6: Classification Report
Reference Case (Imbalanced Dataset)

Cl.	Precision	Recall	F1-Score	Support
P	0.95	0.99	0.97	703
A	0.90	0.66	0.76	255
L	0.93	0.92	0.93	806
N	0.96	0.99	0.98	7500
R	0.99	0.91	0.95	726
f	0.82	0.09	0.16	99
j	0.00	0.00	0.00	23
Accuracy			0.96	10112
Macro avg	0.79	0.65	0.68	10112
Micro avg	0.96	0.96	0.96	10112

Table 7.7: Confusion Matrix (%)
Reference Case (Imbalanced Dataset)

	P	A	L	N	R	f	j
P	98.2	0.14	0.85	0.43	0.00	0.43	0.00
A	0.00	67.1	3.53	27.1	2.35	0.00	0.00
L	0.00	0.00	99.6	0.25	0.00	0.12	0.00
N	0.03	0.07	0.73	98.8	0.31	0.03	0.00
R	0.00	0.14	0.00	2.35	97.5	0.00	0.00
f	5.05	0.00	7.07	20.2	2.02	65.7	0.00
j	0.00	0.00	0.00	73.9	21.7	0.00	4.35

Table 7.8: Classification Report
Case I: Conditional GAN, Raw Gen. Beats

Cl.	Precision	Recall	F1-Score	Support
P	0.95	1.00	0.98	703
A	0.62	0.92	0.74	255
L	0.86	0.99	0.92	806
N	1.00	0.90	0.95	7500
R	0.76	0.99	0.86	726
f	0.35	0.89	0.50	99
j	0.12	0.74	0.20	23
Accuracy			0.92	10112
Macro avg	0.67	0.92	0.74	10112
Micro avg	0.95	0.92	0.93	10112

Table 7.9: Confusion Matrix (%)
Case I: Conditional GAN, Raw Gen. Beats

	P	A	L	N	R	f	j
P	99.9	0.14	0.00	0.00	0.00	0.00	0.00
A	0.78	92.2	0.39	1.18	3.92	0.39	1.18
L	0.12	0.87	98.89	0.00	0.00	0.00	0.12
N	0.24	1.79	1.65	89.75	2.85	2.07	1.65
R	0.14	0.14	0.14	0.14	99.3	0.14	0.00
f	11.2	0.00	0.00	0.00	0.00	88.8	0.00
j	0.00	0.00	0.00	8.70	0.00	17.4	73.9

Table 7.10: Classification Report
Case II: Conditional GAN, Screened Gen. Beats

Cl.	Precision	Recall	F1-Score	Support
P	0.99	0.95	0.97	703
A	0.52	0.96	0.67	255
L	0.91	0.99	0.95	806
N	1.00	0.92	0.96	7500
R	0.86	0.99	0.92	726
f	0.43	0.95	0.59	99
j	0.22	0.78	0.34	23
Accuracy			0.94	10112
Macro avg	0.70	0.93	0.77	10112
Micro avg	0.96	0.94	0.94	10112

Table 7.11: Confusion Matrix (%)
Case II: Conditional GAN, Screened Gen. Beats

	P	A	L	N	R	f	j
P	95.3	1.14	0.14	0.14	0.00	2.99	0.28
A	0.00	96.1	0.39	2.75	0.00	0.78	0.00
L	0.00	0.37	98.5	0.74	0.12	0.25	0.00
N	0.05	2.88	1.00	92.4	1.55	1.27	0.80
R	0.00	0.41	0.00	0.41	98.9	0.00	0.28
f	5.05	0.00	0.00	0.00	0.00	95.0	0.00
j	0.00	0.00	0.00	8.70	0.00	13.0	78.3

Table 7.12: Classification Report
Case III: Unconditional GAN, Raw Gen. Beats

Cl.	Precision	Recall	F1-Score	Support
P	0.98	0.99	0.99	703
A	0.48	0.98	0.64	255
L	0.94	0.99	0.96	806
N	1.00	0.92	0.96	7500
R	0.90	1.00	0.94	726
f	0.40	0.92	0.56	99
j	0.15	0.87	0.25	23
Accuracy			0.93	10112
Macro avg	0.69	0.95	0.76	10112
Micro avg	0.97	0.93	0.94	10112

Table 7.13: Confusion Matrix (%)
Case III: Unconditional GAN, Raw Gen. Beats

	P	A	L	N	R	f	j
P	99.0	0.28	0.00	0.14	0.00	0.57	0.00
A	0.00	97.65	0.39	0.39	0.78	0.39	0.39
L	0.00	0.37	98.9	0.12	0.12	0.50	0.00
N	0.07	3.51	0.69	91.5	1.05	1.65	1.51
R	0.00	0.14	0.00	0.00	99.6	0.00	0.28
f	6.06	0.00	1.01	0.00	1.01	91.9	0.00
j	0.00	0.00	0.00	4.35	4.35	4.35	87.0

Table 7.14: Classification Report
Case IV: Unconditional GAN, Screened

Cl.	Precision	Recall	F1-Score	Support
P	0.93	1.00	0.96	703
A	0.58	0.96	0.72	255
L	0.91	1.00	0.95	806
N	1.00	0.93	0.97	7500
R	0.92	0.99	0.96	726
f	0.48	0.84	0.61	99
j	0.25	0.87	0.39	23
Accuracy			0.95	10112
Macro avg	0.72	0.94	0.79	10112
Micro avg	0.96	0.95	0.95	10112

Table 7.15: Confusion Matrix (%)
Case IV: Unconditional GAN, Screened

	P	A	L	N	R	f	j
P	99.9	0.14	0.00	0.00	0.00	0.00	0.00
A	0.39	96.1	0.00	1.96	1.57	0.00	0.00
L	0.12	0.25	99.5	0.00	0.12	0.00	0.00
N	0.56	2.36	0.99	93.4	0.72	1.20	0.73
R	0.00	0.14	0.00	0.14	99.2	0.00	0.55
f	12.1	0.00	1.01	2.02	0.00	83.8	1.01
j	0.00	0.00	0.00	8.70	0.00	4.35	87.0

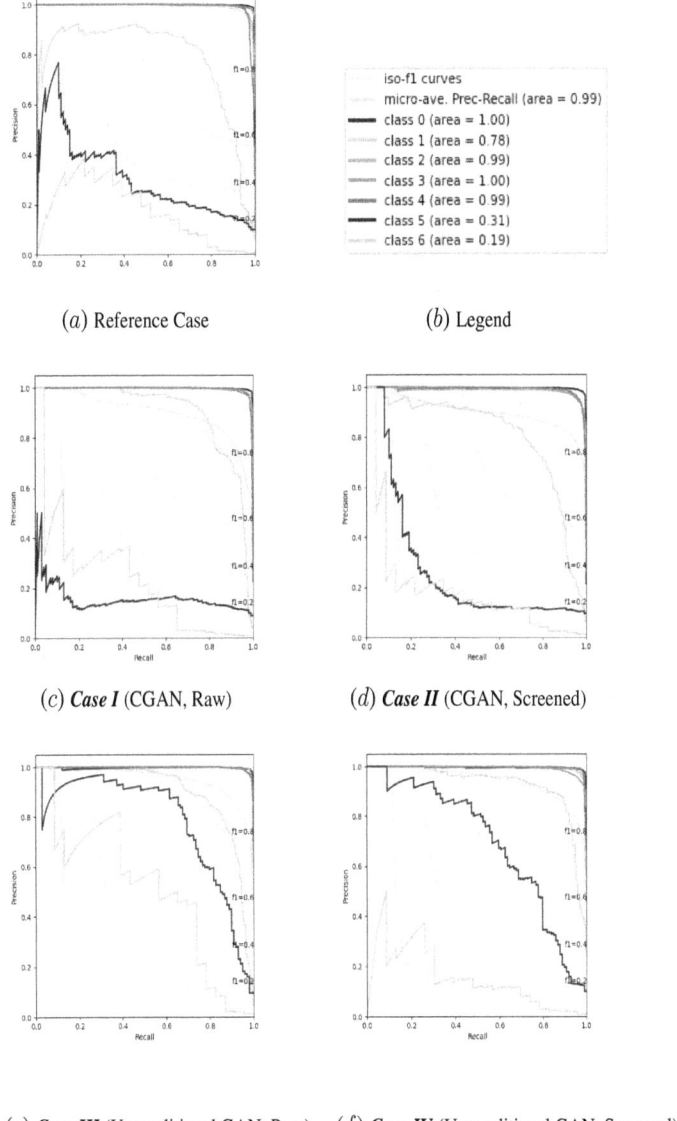

Figure 7.3: Precision-Recall Curves

7.6.5 Net Improvements in True Positives

Another metric that is used in this study is the *total* net improvements in true positives (main diagonals in the confusion matrix). For calculation of this metric *all* the elements on the main diagonal of the confusion matrix in the reference case are subtracted from the corresponding elements in each case and the results are summed up algebraically. For the improvements in *minor classes* the same method has been used, but only minor classes ("i" and "j") are considered. We believe this simple metric, which focuses only on true positives, is more tangible for the purpose of this study, because here we are only interested in those synthetic samples which can be classified correctly. As seen from Table 7.16, *Case III* produces the most improvements in true positives (*total* and *minor-classes*), which is consistent with the other two metrics.

Table 7.16: Net Improvement in True Positives (%)

-	Case I	Case II	Case III	Case IV
Total	111.4	123.3	*134.3*	127.6
Minor-Classes	92.68	103.2	*108.9*	100.8

7.7 Conclusion

In this paper, we developed a conditional AC-WGAN-GP model *in one dimensional form* for the first time and implemented it along with a non-conditional WGAN-GP model to investigate the impact of data augmentation in arrhythmia detection. We employed the two models to generate synthetic heartbeats samples in 7 arrhythmia classes from the MIT-BIH Arrhythmia dataset. Two scenarios have been considered for each model: *(i)* raw data, i.e., all the generated data have been used for augmentation and *(ii)* screened data, i.e., only good-quality generated beats (determined by the DTW distance function) have been used. Thus, four study cases are developed. The state-of-the-art classifier (*EcgResNet34*) is employed to investigate the effectiveness of data augmentation. First, the classifier is trained on the original imbalanced dataset (reference case) and then on the four augmented datasets. Then, the trained classifier in each case is used to classify the same holdout unseen data (test set) and then the classification metrics are compared. The metrics used are *(i)* micro-averaged Precision score, *(ii)* multiclass Precision-Recall graph and *(iii)* the net improvements in the number of true positives (*total* and *minor-class*). We believe that this last metric is the most suitable one for the purpose of this study, because we are interested only in the number of synthetic beats that can be classified correctly. All the three metrics consistently select **Case III**, i.e., unconditional GAN with no screening.

It might seem that screened cases should produce better improvements in true positives as the low-quality beats are already discarded from training set. However, during screening and by discarding some of the generated beats, the distribution changes. Since GAN models implicitly mimic the distribution of the training set in the generated data, the distribution of the generated data would be different from the original real dataset in screened cases. Thus, the augmented set is composed of two sets of data with two different distributions. This would negatively impact the training, optimization and convergence of the parameters of the classifier model.

CHAPTER 8: *(PAPER 3)*
GENERATION OF SYNTHETIC ECG SIGNALS USING PROBABILISTIC DIFFUSION MODELS

8.1 Overview and Contribution

In this paper [3] we present a pipeline to generate $1D$ synthetic ECG signals using $2D$ DDPM. We also investigate the quality of the generated beats by DDPM and compare it with GAN models. To the best of our knowledge, this is the first time that diffusion models are used for the generation of synthetic ECG signals.

The $1D$ ECG time series data are embedded into 3-channel $2D$ data space (similar to RGB image files) using *Gramian Angular Summation/Difference Fields* (GASF/GADF) and *Markov Transition Fields* (MTF) [76] and then the embedded data are fed to the Improved DDPM as image files. DDPM is trained on the embedded data and then sampled to generate embedded $2D$ ECG data which are then de-embedded and transformed back to $1D$ space and ECG time series are reconstructed using the inverse transformations (Figure. 8.1).

Three different settings of DDPM hyper-parameters have been considered as three study cases and the fourth study case is the data generated by the WGAN-GP model. The generated data by the four study cases are compared in terms of the:

- *Quality* (measured by DTW distance function)

- *Distribution* (measured by Maximum Mean Discrepancy, MMD)

- *Authenticity* (measured by the devised authenticity test)

Here, by the *authenticity* of the synthetic beats we mean whether they can replace and function as the real data in a classification test. The data generated by the four study cases are used to train a classifier and the trained classifier is put to test by classifying a binary test set (unseen and real). The following standard classification metrics are used to compare the performance of classification in the four study cases:

- Precision score,

- Area Under Curve (AUC) of Precision-Recall curves (AUC Pr-Re),

- Area Under Curve (AUC) of Receiver Operating Characteristic curves (ROC AUC)

MIT-BIH Arrhythmia dataset [53] [27] is used as the dataset with the adaptive window segmentation (Section 3.9.2). Since this research is the first use of DDPM in ECG generation, we employed DDPM in the unconditional form and focused only on the *Normal Sinus* class to investigate the feasibility of the idea. However, it can be also used in the conditional form for generating synthetic arrhythmia signals in various classes.

3rd Paper:
General Pipeline

- 1D ECG data are mapped into 2D space

- DM is used *as-is* to generate 2D ECG data

- 2D ECG data are mapped back to 1D space

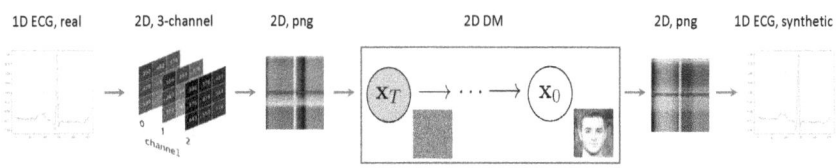

Figure 8.1: Proposed Pipeline

8.3 1D →2D Embedding

Wang et al. [76] proposed a novel embedding framework for mapping time series data from one-dimensional space into two-dimensional space, which enabled the utilization of computer vision techniques *as-is* for time series analysis. First, they map the ECG time series from Cartesian to polar coordinates. Then, they use *Gramian Angular Summation/Difference Fields* (GASF/GADF) and *Markov Transition Fields* (MTF) to build 3 separate $2D$ matrix embeddings of the time series and finally put them together to create a 3-channel $2D$ image file similar to an RGB image file. The proposed pipeline in this study (Fig. 8.1) has been used only for the DDPM, whereas in the WGAN-GP model, all the data (training and generated) and the model itself are in the $1D$ space and no embedding was necessary.

8.4 Polar Coordinate Representation of ECG

ECG time series are one-dimensional, vector-like data, $X = \{x_1, x_2, \ldots, x_N\}$, which represent the time-progression of the induced voltage to the electrode caused by the motion of the electrical impulse generated by the sinoatrial (SA) node in the heart. When normalized and rescaled, ($\tilde{X}$), all the timestep values in $\tilde{X} = \{\tilde{x}_1, \tilde{x}_2, \ldots, \tilde{x}_N\}$ are between -1 and 1, i.e., $\tilde{x}_i \in [-1, 1]$ for $i = 0, \ldots, N$. Thus, each value can be interpreted as the cosine of an imaginary angle $\varphi_i \in [0, \pi]$ [76]:

$$\tilde{x}_i = \cos(\varphi_i) \quad \text{and} \quad \varphi_i = \arccos(\tilde{x}_i) \tag{8.1}$$

Thus, the polar coordinates of mapped data will be (Fig. 8.2):

$$\begin{cases} \varphi_i = \arccos(\tilde{x}_i) & -1 \leq \tilde{x}_i \leq 1 \\ r_i = \frac{i}{N} & i \in [1, N] \end{cases} \tag{8.2}$$

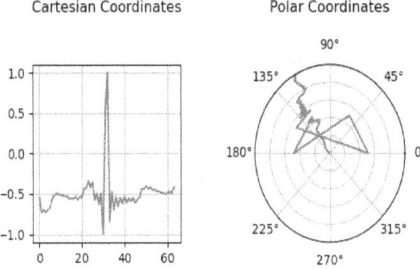

Figure 8.2: *Normal Sinus* ECG Beat in Cartesian and Polar Coordinates

This mapping is *bijective* (one-to-one correspondence) as $\cos(\varphi)$ is monotonic when $\varphi \in [0, \pi]$. Therefore, the forward as well as reverse mappings are unique. Also, the temporal relations of the timesteps are preserved in the mapping.

8.5 Gramian Angular Fields (GASF/GADF)

After transformation into polar coordinates, the *Gramian Summation Angular Field* (GASF) and the *Gramian Difference Angular Field* (GADF) matrices are defined [76]:

$$GASF = \begin{bmatrix} \cos\left(\frac{\varphi_1}{2} + \frac{\varphi_1}{2}\right) & \cdots & \cos\left(\frac{\varphi_1}{2} + \frac{\varphi_N}{2}\right) \\ \vdots & \ddots & \vdots \\ \cos\left(\frac{\varphi_N}{2} + \frac{\varphi_1}{2}\right) & \cdots & \cos\left(\frac{\varphi_N}{2} + \frac{\varphi_N}{2}\right) \end{bmatrix} \quad (8.3)$$

$$GADF = \begin{bmatrix} \cos\left(\frac{\varphi_1}{2} - \frac{\varphi_1}{2}\right) & \cdots & \cos\left(\frac{\varphi_1}{2} - \frac{\varphi_N}{2}\right) \\ \vdots & \ddots & \vdots \\ \cos\left(\frac{\varphi_N}{2} - \frac{\varphi_1}{2}\right) & \cdots & \cos\left(\frac{\varphi_N}{2} - \frac{\varphi_N}{2}\right) \end{bmatrix} \quad (8.4)$$

GASF and GADF are in fact quasi-Gramian matrices because the defined *cos()* functions do not satisfy the linear property in the inner-product space, however, they do preserve the temporal dependency of the timesteps in the time series [76]. Additionally, the main diagonal of GASF can be used directly in the de-embedding to reconstruct the original time series in the Cartesian coordinates by Eq. 8.1, as *cos()* is monotonic when $\varphi_i \in [0, \pi]$. In GASF/GADF embedding, half-angles are used because with the full-angles, the mapping in the de-embedding will not be unique ($\cos(2\theta) = 2\cos^2(\theta) - 1 \longrightarrow \cos(\theta) = \pm\frac{1}{2}\sqrt{\cos(2\theta) + 1}$).

8.6 Markov Transition Fields (MTF)

GASF and GADF capture the *static* information in the time series elements without any notion on the *dynamic* information, i.e., how the values in timesteps change in time progression. In contrast, MTF captures the *dynamic* information by setting up some Q quantile bins and assigning each x_i to its corresponding bin q_i where $i \in [1, Q]$. For any pair of x_i and x_j, with the corresponding bins q_i and q_j, M_{ij} in *Matrix Transition Field* (MTF) denotes the probability of transitioning from q_i to q_j. Thus, the MTF matrix takes into account the *temporal positions* as well as *temporal changes* of the timesteps in the time series. The main diagonal in the MTF matrix represents the probability of transitioning from the quantile at timestep i to itself (self-transition probability) [76]:

$$GTF = \begin{bmatrix} M_{11} & \cdots & M_{1N} \\ \vdots & \ddots & \vdots \\ M_{N1} & \cdots & M_{NN} \end{bmatrix} \qquad (8.5)$$

8.7 2D →1D De-embedding

After the diffusion model is trained on the $2D$ embedded data, the trained model is sampled to generate synthetic $2D$ 3-channel ECG data. Since the elements on the main diagonal of the GASF channel of the generated data consist only of the univariate data, $\bar{X} = \{\cos(\bar{\varphi}_1), \ldots, \cos(\bar{\varphi}_N)\}$, we can de-embed the generated $2D$ data back into $1D$ space (i.e., reconstruct the time series) very easily by using Eq. 8.1, given that the mapping is bijective.

8.8 Precision or Recall

In this study we intend to maximize the number of true positives (TP) and at the same time minimize the number of false positives (FP). Thus, $\frac{FP}{TP}$ is to be minimized. Therefore, Precision score ($Pr = \frac{TP}{TP+FP} = \frac{1}{1+FP/TP}$) relates to the purpose of this study more than the Recall score ($Re = \frac{TP}{TP+FN} = \frac{1}{1+FN/TP}$), as in the abundance of the generated data, it is immaterial if some of the *good* samples are overlooked (false negatives).

8.9 Area Under Precision-Recall Curve (AUC Pr-Re)

One of the metrics used to evaluate the performance of binary classification is the area under the Precision-Recall plot. This plot captures the trade-off between the two scores at different (rather than at one single) thresholds. First, in the classification of the whole set of the test data, $Pr = \frac{TP}{TP+FP}$ is plotted against $Re = \frac{TP}{TP+FN}$ when the threshold of classification probability is varied from zero to one. Then the area under the curve of the plot is measured. The area is equal to 1 for a perfect classification [33].

8.10 Area Under Receiver Operator Curve (AUC ROC)

Receiver Operator Curve (ROC) is the plot of $TPR = \frac{TP}{TP+FN}$ against $FPR = \frac{FP}{FP+TN}$. AUC ROC score is a metric which measures the trade-off between TPR and FPR when the threshold of the *classification probability* is varied from zero to one. A higher AUC ROC value indicates a better classification model [33].

8.11 Authenticity or Equivalency of Generated Beats

One of the metrics we used in our comparison is the *authenticity* or *equivalency* test, in which the generated beats are *equivalents* to the real beat. In other words, they are checked whether they can function as and replace the *real* beats in a classification task. This investigation is done via the so-called *classification* or *authenticity* test. The objective of this binary classification test is to distinguish Normal beats from the anomaly (here we picked the typical Class L as the anomaly).

First, the state-of-the-art classifier (ResNet34) is trained on a totally balanced and all-real training set consisting of two classes: N (Normal Beat) and L (Left Bundle Branch Block Beat) with $7,000$ samples in each class. The trained classifier is put to test on an unseen test set and the classification metrics are recorded. This is the *reference case*, and any other study case is compared with this case (Table 8.1). Then, the *compromised case* is formed by imbalancing the training set purposely by reducing the number of samples in N class down to 350. The performance of the classification of the compromised case, which has been made poor intentionally, is recorded. Then, the imbalanced training set is augmented/balanced by the synthetic beats in each of the study cases and the classifier is trained on them. Since the training set is augmented/balanced, the classification performance improves significantly relative to the compromised case. The case which produces the best improvements in the classification metrics has produced the most authentic synthetic beats (Table 8.1). The same test set is used in all cases: 1000 samples of unseen real data in each class with no synthetic beats.

Table 8.1: Authenticity or Equivalency Test Training Set Supports

Cases	Train Set Class N	Train Set Class L
Reference (Balanced, all real)	7000 r	7000 r
Compromised (Imbalanced)	350 r	7000 r
Augmented with case 00	350 r + 6650 s	7000 r
Augmented with case 01	350 r + 6650 s	7000 r
Augmented with case 02	350 r + 6650 s	7000 r
Augmented with case GAN	350 r + 6650 s	7000 r

r: *Real Beat*   s: *Synthetically Generated Beat*

8.11.1 Classifier: ECGResNet34

ResNet34 [35] is the state-of-the-art tool used in the classification of images. It has 34 layers and incorporates *residual* building blocks. Each block is comprised of two 3×3 convolutional layers with a residual stream [35], which reduces the risk of gradient vanishing/exploding. It is pretrained on the ImageNet dataset (more than $100,000$ images in 200 classes). We used its $1D$ implementation [48] for our classification test.

8.12 Experimental Setup

8.12.1 WGAN-GP Model Design

The architectures of the generator and the critic in the WGAN-GP model are comprised of building blocks that are repeated multiple times (Table 8.2). The details of the architectures of the generator and the critic are shown in Table 8.3.

Table 8.2: WGAN-GP Building Blocks

Layer	Generator	Critic
1	ConvTranspose1d [1]	ConvTranspose1d [1]
2	BatchNorm1d	InstanceNorm1d
3	ReLU	LeakyReLU

[1]: *kernel size = 4, stride = 2, padding = 1*

Table 8.3: WGAN-GP Architecture

Layer	Generator	Critic
Input	$16 \times 100 \times 1$	$16 \times 1 \times 64$
1	Block	Vonv1d, LeakyReLU
2	Block	Block
3	Block	Block
4	Block	Block
5	ConvTranspose1d	Conv1d
6	FC	FC
7	tanh	-
Output	$16 \times 1 \times 64$	$16 \times 1 \times 1$

8.12.2 Improved DDPM Model Design

Improved DDPM [56] has been used *as-is* as the diffusion model. Codes of the DDPM are taken from [56] (https://github.com/openai/improved-diffusion).

8.12.3 Platform and GitHub Code

The training of and sampling from the DDPMs are done on the Arc (the HPC cluster at the University of Texas at San Antonio (UTSA)). Currently, Arc can run programs with two V-100 GPUs on each node. For this study, one node from the cluster with two parallel GPUs has been used.

For the rest of the computations, a desktop and a laptop have been used: a Dell Alienware desktop with Intel i9-9900k at 3.6 GHz (8 cores, 16 threads) microprocessor, 64 GB RAM, and NVIDIA GeForce RTX 2080 Ti graphics card with 24 GB RAM, and a personal Dell G7 laptop with an Intel i7-8750H at 2.2 GHz (6 cores, 12 threads) microprocessor, 20 GB of RAM, and NVIDIA GeForce 1060 MaxQ graphics card with 6 GB. Our codes are available on the GitHub page of the paper (https://github.com/mah533/Synthetic-ECG-Signal-Generation-using-Probabilistic-Diffusion-Models).

8.12.4 DM, GAN and Real Study Cases

Three different hyperparameter settings for the Improved DDPM have been considered which are shown in Table 8.4. The rest of the parameters are the same for all cases.

Table 8.4: DM Case Studies

Cases	Learn Sigma	Noise Schedule	Use KL [1]	Schedule Sampler
00	False	Linear	False	Uniform
01	True	Cosine	True	Uniform
02	True	Cosine	True	loss second moment

1: *Kullback-Leibeler (KL) Divergence*

The above three study cases have been compared to the 4th case, which is the synthetic ECG beats generated by the WGAN-GP. Since the ultimate goal is to generate realistic synthetic beats that resemble and function like real beats as closely as possible, an additional *case (rl)* is considered for reference, in which real beats have been used instead of synthetic ones in the corresponding comparison.

8.13 Results

Samples of the generated synthetic ECG signals ($1D$ and $2D$) are shown in the Figure 8.3. The aforementioned four case studies are compared by the *quality*, *distribution* and *authenticity* of the generated beats in each case.

8.13.1 Quality

When discussing the quality of the beats, we refer to how much the generated synthetic beats resemble the real ones in appearance and morphology. For assessing the quality of the heartbeats

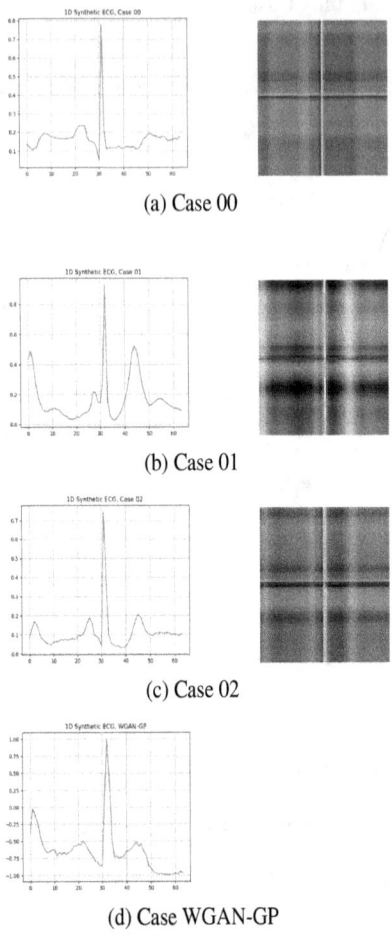

(a) Case 00

(b) Case 01

(c) Case 02

(d) Case WGAN-GP

Figure 8.3: Samples of Synthetically Generated ECG Signals

quantitatively, *the average distances of the generated beats from a randomly selected template* is measured using two distance functions (AKA similarity measures): Dynamic Time Warping (DTW) and Fréchet distance functions. Both distance functions consistently show that the generated beats by the WGAN-GP model are by far closer to the reference case (rl), in terms of quality (Table 8.5).

Table 8.5: Quality of Generated Beats

Cases	Ave. DTW Distance	Ave. Fréchet Distance
00	6.67	1.074
01	6.95	1.117
02	6.36	1.042
GAN	2.12	0.723
Real (rl)	2.09	0.718

8.13.2 Distribution

Maximum Mean Discrepancy (MMD) is a kernel based statistical tool to measure the distance between two *distributions* (Eq. 8.6) [30]. To compare the distributions of generated beat sets, equal number of samples (7000, i.e., the total number of generated beats) from the real data (rl) and the generated data in each case are selected randomly, ($m = n = 7000$) and the MMD value between them is measured utilizing the linear kernel. For reference, the MMD value between two disjoint sets of real samples is shown as well (Table 8.6).

$$MMD^2(p,q) = \mathbb{E}_{x,x'}\left[k\left(x_i, x'_j\right)\right] - 2\mathbb{E}_{x,y}\left[k\left(x_i, y_j\right)\right] + \mathbb{E}_{y,y'}\left[k\left(y_i, y'_j\right)\right] =$$

$$\frac{1}{m(m-1)}\sum_{i=1}^{m}\sum_{j\neq i}^{m} k(x_i, x_j) - \frac{2}{mn}\sum_{i=1}^{m}\sum_{j=1}^{n} k(x_i, x_j) + \frac{1}{n(n-1)}\sum_{i=1}^{n}\sum_{j\neq i}^{n} k(y_i, y_j) \quad (8.6)$$

Table 8.6: MMD Value of Synthetic and Real Beats

Cases	00-rl	01-rl	02-rl	GAN-rl	rl-rl
MMD	39.8	44	35.9	1.00	0.0

In terms of the distribution of the generated beats, the WGAN-GP model generates beats much closer to the real beats than the diffusion models do.

8.13.3 Authenticity or Equivalency

Here we quantitatively measure if the generated beats are *equivalent* to the real beats, in other words, how much the generated beats can replace (i.e., function as) the real ones in a classification test. The metrics used for the authenticity tests are: *(i)* Average Precision Scores, *(ii)* the Area Under the Curve (AUC) of the Precision-Recall Curves, as well as *(iii)* the AUC of the Receiver Operating Characteristic curves (AUC ROC score).

The Average Precision scores show that WGAN-GP model outperforms the DDPM in correctly classifying the beats, minimizing FP and maximizing TP. It should be noted that micro- and macro-averages are the same as the test set is balanced (Table 8.7).

Table 8.7: Authenticity of Generated Beats

Cases	Ave Precision	PRC [1] AUC [2] Score	ROC [3] AUC Score
00	0.90	0.95	0.96
01	0.55	0.68	0.63
02	0.76	0.76	0.81
GAN	0.96	0.99	0.99
Real (rl)	0.98	1.00	1.00

1: *Precision-Recall Curve*
2: *Area Under Curve*
3: *Receiver Operating Characteristic Curve*

Confusion Matrix

The elements on the main diagonal of the confusion matrix show the percentage of number of times the beats are classified correctly. Again, the synthetic beats generated by the WGAN-GP model behave much more like real beats than the beats generated by DDPM do.

Table 8.8: Confusion Matrices (all values are in %)

	Pred. N	Pred. L
Real N	85.7	14.3
Real L	5.4	94.6

(a) Case 00

	Pred. N	Pred. L
Real N	37.1	62.9
Real L	28.2	71.8

(b) Case 01

	Pred. N	Pred. L
Real N	73.6	26.4
Real L	21.0	79.0

(c) Case 02

	Pred. N	Pred. L
Real N	93.9	6.1
Real L	1.8	98.2

(d) Case GAN

	Pred. N	Pred. L
Real N	99.4	0.6
Real L	3.4	96.6

(e) Case real

Precision - Recall Curves

The Precision-Recall curves' Area Under Curve, (PR AUC), score is a better metric than the Average Precision score, which is calculated at only one threshold. By checking the Precision-Recall curves visually, it can be seen that the WGAN-GP model (Figure 8.4 (d)) produces a graph very close to the real case (Figure 8.4 (e)). However, case 00 has the best PR curve among the DDPM cases (Figure 8.4 (a)). Also, the Precision-Recall AUC score (Table 8.7) confirms the visual check. The same argument holds for the ROC AUC score.

8.14 Discussion

In a typical classification task, since there is no need to map the data back into their original space, no *invertibility* condition is required for the embedding. Threrfor, $1D$ time series can be embedded into $2D$ space by any embedding technique, such as [28]. As long as there is one *and only one* corresponding element in the embedded space, and no two datapoints in the original space have the same mapped datapoint in the destination space (i.e., *injective* mapping), mapping is acceptable.

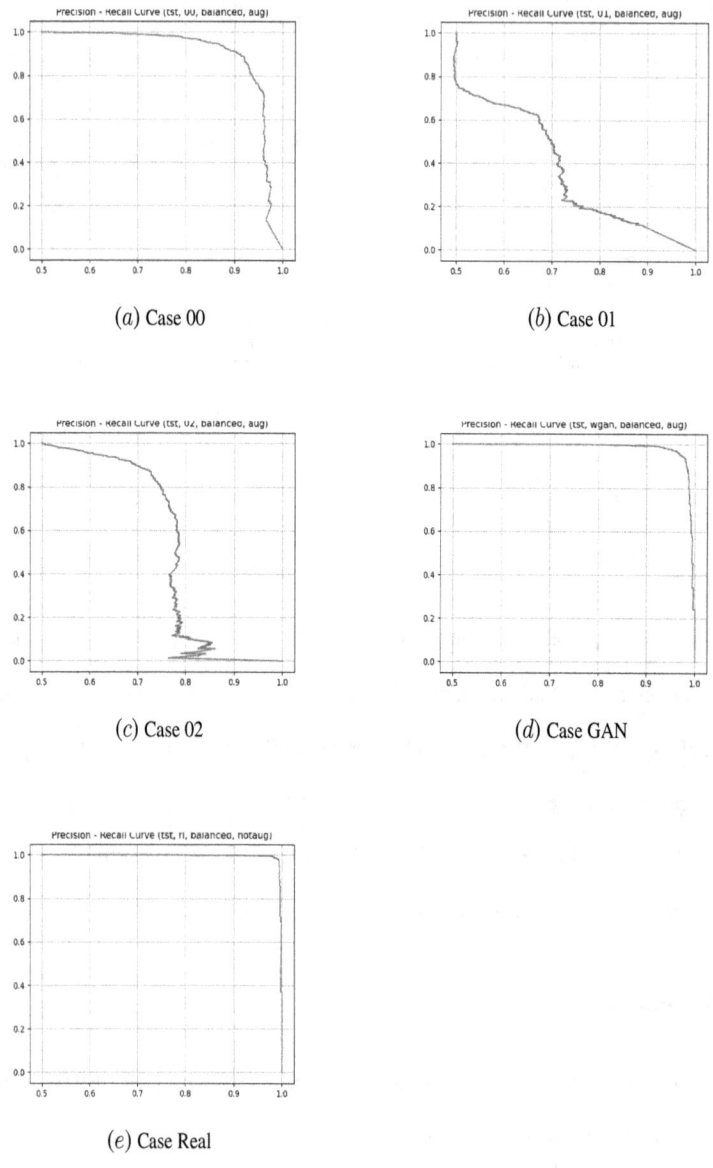

Figure 8.4: Precision-Recall Curves

However, in generation tasks, the generated data must be de-embedded and mapped back into the original space. Therefore, the mapping must be *bijective*. That is why the spectrograms are useful in classification tasks but not in generation tasks.

Each ECG beat in our dataset has 64 timesteps. Therefore with the WGAN-GP model, each time, 64 pieces of information are generated per heartbeat, 100% of which from the user's perspective are *useful information*. Whereas in DDPM, $3 \times 64 \times 64 = 12,288$ pieces of information are generated per beat, from which only 64 pieces (5.2%) are useful/extracted and the rest are discarded. In the training of the deep learning models, the optimization process finds the optimum values of the trainable parameters in a way that each piece of the generated information are in some certain neighborhood. The total error in the loss function is *typically* comprised of 64 elements in the WGAN-GP and $12,288$ elements in DDPM per beat. Thus, a tighter neighborhood in WGAN-GP (closer to the real beats) and a more relaxed one in DDPM is quite natural.

8.15 Conclusion

8.15.1 what we did

In this paper, we presented a pipeline to generate synthetic $1D$ ECG time series using the $2D$ probabilistic diffusion model (Improved DDPM).

8.15.2 Why we did it

With the remarkable success of $2D$ computer vision models, specifically the Improved DDPM and its superiority to the GAN models [56] [17]) and the widespread availability of their pretrained version, it makes sense to apply them to $1D$ time series. One of the benefits of the processing of the data in $2D$ space is providing additional data augmentation techniques (such as flipping, rotation, and mirroring), which are helpful specifically in classification tasks.

8.15.3 How we did it

In this study, we used unconditional models and used only the N class (*Normal Sinus Beat*) from the MIT-BIH Arrhythmia dataset [53] [27]. The general pipeline used in this study is shown in Figure. 8.1. First, the $1D$ ECG time series are transformed into the polar coordinates. Then, they are embedded into the 3-channel $2D$ space, similar to RGB image files. *Gramian Summation/Difference Fields* (GASF/GADF) and *Markov Transition Field* (MTF) are used to produce the three $2D$ matrices, which are then put together to form one single image file for each beat. The Improved DDPM model [56] is trained and sampled to generate $2D$ ECG signals, which are then de-embedded to reconstruct a $1D$ ECG signal. The generated data by DDPM are in 3 study cases with 3 different settings in hyperparameters. They are compared to the synthetically generated data by WGAN-GP, as well as to the *real beats*, to see how close the cases are to reality, since the ultimate goal is to generate realistic synthetic ECG beats. The comparison is done in terms of the *quality*, *distribution*, and *authenticity* of the data (i.e., up to what extent they can replace the *real* beats in data augmentation for classification tasks).

8.15.4 results summary

The results show that the synthetic beats generated by the WGAN-GP model are consistently closer to the real beats than the beats from DDPM, in all cases and by all the metrics used. The average distances of the beats from a template (measured by the DTW and Fréchet Distance functions) as well as the distribution of generated beats (measured by MMD) respectively reveal that the *quality* and the *distribution* of the beats from the WGAN-GP are much closer to the corresponding real ones than those of the DDPM. For quantifying the *authenticity* of the generated beats, we used a classification test using the-state-of-the-art classifier ResNet34 [35] and several standard classification metrics, namely average precision score, AUC of Precision-Recall curves, and AUC of ROC curves, all of which constantly show that the WGAN-GP model outperforms the Improved DDPM in this regard.

8.16 Limitations and Future Works

The Improved DDPM [56] developed by OpenAI is a $2D$ model, i.e., the input/output data and the processing, are in $2D$ space and it has been used in this study *as-is* with almost no changes. We proposed the pipeline in Figure 8.1 for this application, where the $1D$ ECG data are mapped into a $2D$ space, converted into image files, and fed to a DDPM model. The processing takes place in the $2D$ space and the generated $2D$ data is de-embedded back into $1D$ space, where the $1D$ ECG data are reconstructed, whereas the WGAN-GP model developed and used in this study is inherently $1D$, i.e., the input/output data and the processing are all in $1D$ space, with no embedding necessary. It should be emphasized that the conclusions drawn here apply only to the setting and the pipeline used in this research, and the results might be different in any other setting.

Although the probabilistic diffusion model is being applied to images and $2D$ data mostly, the general concept can be applied to $1D$ data as well, i.e., the model can take $1D$ data, perform the noising/denoising processes in $1D$ space, and generate synthetic data in $1D$ without any embedding. In this case, the model would be a better representative of the diffusion concept and the comparison would be more realistic.

CHAPTER 9: FUTURE DIRECTIONS

9.1 Diffusion-GAN Hybrid Model

The two main categories of deep generative algorithms are: *(1)* likelihood-based models and *(2)* Adversarial Network Models. Investigation of the loss function of the likelihood-based models (e.g., VAE, Eq. 4.4) reveals that the loss function makes the distribution of the data generated by the parameterized DL model as close as possible to the original real dataset. This means that during the optimization step of the training, parameters of the model are optimized to fulfill this requirement rather than solely focusing on the *quality* or distance of the generated data from the real data. On the other hand, the loss function of adversarial networks (Eq. 4.13) emphasizes the average (expected value) of the generated data, where the focus lies on the generated data themselves rather than their distributions.

Diffusion models, which belong to the likelihood-based category, are known to be sluggish due to theoretical restrictions on the magnitude of the added/removed noise [56]. Therefore, there exists a trilemma in these categories of generative algorithms [80]:

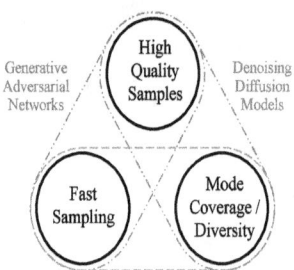

Figure 9.1: Generative learning trilemma

The natural question that arises here is: *is it possible to combine GAN and DM in a way that both the speed of GAN and the mode coverage of likelihood-based models are exploited?*

There have been several successful attempts [75, 80]. One of the architectures is shown in

Figure 9.2 [80]:

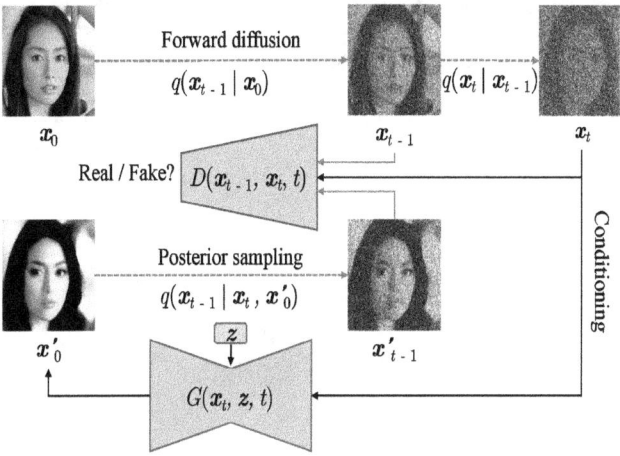

Figure 9.2: Diffusion-GAN Hybrid Architecture

In this concept, the noisy version of the *real* image and the noisy version of the *fake* image are compared (at the same timesteps) in the discriminator. When the discriminator cannot distinguish between the two, the training is accomplished, and the generator is ready to generate synthetic data. Note that the addition of the random variable z converts the process from deterministic to stochastic, so that, at each sampling attempt, a different image is generated.

The application of this concept to the generation of synthetic ECG signals, and comparing the proposed metrics (quality, distribution, and authenticity or equivalence) with other deep generative algorithms seems to be a good candidate for a research topic.

9.2 Cryo-ET/EM

Cryogenic Electron Microscopy or Electron Tomography (Cryo-EM/ET) is one of the emerging technologies (Figure 9.3) that is on the brink of revolutionizing molecular and structural biology [49]. It produces electron-sized resolution images from the diffraction of the electron beams radiated to an extremely thin cellular tissues, identifying organelles and macromolecules within the cells, without requiring any template or additional information (size, conformational stage, ...).

This technology utilizes techniques similar to the object detection YOLO technique to identify organelles [63, 85]. However, the technology faces some challenges such ad the low SNR of the produced images, which is caused by the restriction on the electron beam dose. High doses might be detrimental to the tissue, and there are also physical constraints on the maximum/minimum rotation angle of the grid (tissue) [72].

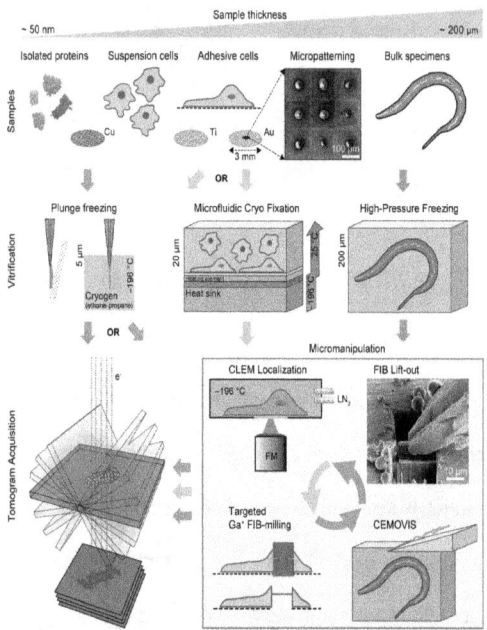

Figure 9.3: Cryo ET/EM Technology

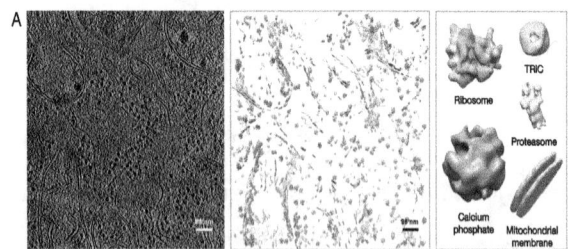

Figure 9.4: Cryo ET/EM 3D Image Reconstruction

One of the applications of deep generative algorithms is denoising images, including biomedical images (e.g., [44, 65, 89]). A potential area of research would involve devising new DL techniques to denoise tomograms and sub-tomograms generated by Cryo-EM/ET.

www.ingramcontent.com/pod-product-compliance
Lightning Source LLC
LaVergne TN
LVHW011946070526
838202LV00054B/4819